BIOTERRORISM AND PUBLIC HEALTH

BIOTERRORISM AND PUBLIC HEALTH

VITALI B. MELLEHOVITCH
EDITOR

Nova Science Publishers, Inc.
New York

Coordinating Editor: Tatiana Shohov
Senior Editors: Susan Boriotti and Donna Dennis
Office Manager: Annette Hellinger
Graphics: Wanda Serrano and Matt Dallow
Editorial Production: Alexandra Columbus, Maya Columbus, Alexis Klestov, Vladimir Klestov, Matthew Kozlowski and Lorna Loperfido
Circulation: Ave Maria Gonzalez, Vera Popovic, Luis Aviles, Sean Corkery, Raymond Davis, Melissa Diaz, Meagan Flaherty, Magdalena Nuñez, Marlene Nuñez, Jeannie Pappas and Frankie Punger
Communications and Acquisitions: Serge P. Shohov
Marketing: Cathy DeGregory

Library of Congress Cataloging-in-Publication Data
Available upon request

ISBN 1-59033-941-X

400 Oser Ave, Suite 1600
Hauppauge, New York 11788-3619
Tele. 631-231-7269 Fax 631-231-8175
e-mail: Novascience@earthlink.net
Web Site: http://www.novapublishers.com

Printed in the United States of America

CONTENTS

FOREWORD

On June 12, 2002, the President signed into law the Public Health Security and bioterrorism Preparedness and Response Act of 2002 (P.L. 107-188, H.R. 3448), which is intended to bolster the nation's ability to respond effectively to bioterrorist threats and other public health emergencies. Chapter one provides an overview and legislative history of P.L. 107-188, followed by a detailed side-by-side comparison of the act's provisions with preexisting law. Appendix A lists, by committee, all the bioterrorism-related hearings held in the 107th Congress prior to enactment of P.L. 107-188. It provides a brief overview and legislative history of P.L. 107-188, followed by a detailed side-by-side comparison of the act's provisions with preexisting law.

Chapter two summarizes H.R. 3448 and S. 1765 and provides a side-by-side comparison of the provisions in each bill and in current law before it became P.L. 107-188.

To better understand the preparedness gaps that exist, as well as the disparate functions and agencies that define public health in this country, CRS, in conjunction with George Washington University's National Health Policy Forum, convened a seminar on October 26, 2001, entitled, The U.S. Health Care system: Are State and Local Officials Prepared for Bioterrorism? How Should the Federal Government Assist? Chapter three summarizes presentations made at the seminar.

Federal research and preparedness activities related to bioterrorism center on detecting of such agents; developing new or improved vaccines, antibiotics, and antivirals; and developing performance standards for emergency response equipment. Preparedness activities include: (1) increasing federal, state, and local response capabilities; (2) developing response teams; (3) increasing the availability of medical treatments; (4) participating in and sponsoring exercises; (5) aiding victims; and (6) providing support at special events, such as presidential inaugurations and Olympic games. To coordinate their activities, federal agencies are developing interagency response plans, participating in various interagency work groups, and entering into formal agreements with each other to share resources and capabilities. In chapters four and five the GAO found that coordination of federal terrorism research, preparedness, and response programs is fragmented, raising concerns about the ability of states and localities to respond to a bioterrorist attack. These concerns include poor state and local planning and the lack of hospital participation in training on terrorism and emergency response planning.

Following the bioterrorist events of the fall of 2001, there has been concern that the nation may not be prepared to respond to a major public health threat, such as the current outbreak of Severe Acute Respiratory Syndrome (SARS). Whether a disease outbreak occurs naturally or is due to the intentional release of a harmful biological agent by a terrorist, much of the initial response would occur at the local level, particularly hospitals and their emergency departments. Efforts to plan for worldwide influenza pandemics are useful for understanding public health preparedness for other large-scale outbreaks. In chapter six the GAO examines (1) the preparedness of state and local public health agencies and organizations for responding to a large-scale infectious disease outbreak, (2) the preparedness of hospitals for responding to a large-scale infectious disease outbreak, and (3) federal and state efforts to prepare for an influenza pandemic.

In the fall of 2001, letters containing anthrax spores were mailed to news media personnel and congressional officials, leading to the first cases of anthrax infection related to an intentional release of anthrax in the United States. Outbreaks of anthrax infection were concentrated in six locations, or epicenters, in the country. An examination of the public health response to the anthrax incidents provides an important opportunity to apply lessons learned from that experience to enhance the nation's preparedness for bioterrorism. Because of its interest in bioterrorism preparedness, Congress asked GAO to review the public health response to the anthrax incidents. Specifically, in chapter seven the GAO determines (1) what was learned from the experience that could help improve public health preparedness at the local and state levels and (2) what was learned that could help improve public health preparedness at the federal level and what steps have been taken to make those improvements.

Chapter 1

PUBLIC HEALTH SECURITY AND BIOTERRORISM PREPAREDNESS AND RESPONSE ACT: PROVISIONS AND CHANGES TO PREEXISTING LAW*

C. Stephen Redhead, Donna U. Vogt and Mary E. Tiemann

SUMMARY

Last fall's anthrax attacks, though small in scale compared to the scenarios envisioned by bioterrorism experts, strained the public health system and raised concern that the nation is insufficiently prepared to respond to bioterrorist attacks. Improving public health preparedness and response capacity offers protection not only from bioterrorist attacks, but also from naturally occurring public health emergencies.

On June 12, 2002, the President signed into law the Public Health Security and Bioterrorism Preparedness and Response Act of 2002 (P.L. 107-188, H.R. 3448), which is intended to bolster the nation's ability to respond effectively to bioterrorist threats and other public health emergencies. The act builds on the programs and authorities established in Title III of the Public Health Service (PHS) Act by the Public Health Threats and Emergencies Act of 2000 (P.L. 106-505, Title I).

P.L. 107-188 is a 5-year authorization bill, which calls for a total of $2.4 billion in funding in FY2002, $2.0 billion in FY2003, and such sums as may be necessary for the remaining years. The act authorizes the Secretary of Health and Human Services (HHS) to upgrade and renovate facilities at the Centers for Disease Control and Prevention (CDC), purchase smallpox vaccine, expand the national stockpile of drugs, vaccines, and other emergency medical supplies, and provide grants to state and local governments and hospitals to improve preparedness and planning. The Secretaries of HHS and Agriculture are required to register and regulate facilities that handle potentially dangerous biological agents.

* Excerpted from CRS Report RL31263.

The anti-bioterrorism legislation also includes provisions to protect the nation's food and drug supply and enhance agricultural security, including new regulatory powers for the Food and Drug Administration (FDA) to block the importation of unsafe foods. To protect the drinking water supply, the act requires community water systems to conduct vulnerability assessments and develop emergency response plans. P.L. 107-188 also reauthorizes the Prescription Drug Use Fee Act through FY2007.

INTRODUCTION

The September 11, 2001 terrorist attacks and the subsequent deliberate release of anthrax spores in the mail have focused policymakers' attention on the preparedness and response capability of the U.S. public health system. Though small in scale compared to the scenarios envisioned by bioterrorism experts and played out in recent government exercises, the recent anthrax attacks strained the public health system and exposed weaknesses at the federal, state, and local levels. Many bioterrorism experts believe that had those responsible for the anthrax attacks employed a more sophisticated delivery mechanism or released a deadly communicable biological agent such as smallpox, the health care system may have been overwhelmed.

Bioterrorism poses a unique challenge to the medical care and public health systems. Unlike an explosion or chemical attack, which results in immediate and visible casualties, the public health impact of a biological attack can unfold gradually over time. Until a sufficient number of people arrive at emergency rooms and doctors' offices complaining of similar illnesses, there may be no sign that an attack has taken place. The speed and accuracy with which doctors and laboratories reach the correct diagnoses and report their findings to public health authorities has a direct impact on the number of people who become ill and the number that die. The nation's ability to respond to a bioterrorist attack, therefore, depends crucially on the state of preparedness of its medical care systems and public health infrastructure.

Public health experts have for years complained about the deterioration of the public health system through neglect and lack of funding. They warn that the nation is ill-equipped and insufficiently prepared to respond to a bioterrorist attack. For example, they point out that there are too few medical personnel trained to spot biological attacks, a shortage of sophisticated laboratories to identify the agents, and inadequate supplies of drugs and vaccines to counteract the threat. They also contend that inadequate plans exist for setting up quarantines and emergency facilities to handle the sick and infectious victims. Improving public health preparedness and response capacity offers protection not only from bioterrorist attacks, but also from naturally occurring public health emergencies. Public health officials are increasingly concerned about our exposure and susceptibility to infectious disease and food-borne illness because of global travel, ubiquitous food imports, and the evolution of antibiotic-resistant pathogens.

On June 12, 2002, the President signed into law the Public Health Security and Bioterrorism Preparedness and Response Act of 2002 (P.L. 107-188, H.R. 3448), which is intended to bolster the nation's ability to respond effectively to bioterrorist threats and other public health emergencies. This chapter provides a brief overview and legislative history of P.L. 107-188, followed by a detailed side-by-side comparison of the act's provisions with preexisting law. Appendix A lists, by committee, all the bioterrorism-related hearings held in the 107th Congress prior to enactment of P.L. 107-188. In most cases, hearing testimony is available on the committee Web sites. Appendix B provides a list of bioterrorism-related Web sites.

PUBLIC HEALTH SECURITY AND BIOTERRORISM PREPAREDNESS AND RESPONSE ACT

Legislative History

Representatives Tauzin (R-LA) and Dingell (D-MI) introduced the Public Health Security and Bioterrorism Response Act (H.R. 3448) on December 11, 2001. The bill was immediately considered under suspension of the rules and passed by the House the following day on a vote of 418-2. H.R. 3448 built on the provisions of a bipartisan Senate bill, the Bioterrorism Preparedness Act (S. 1765), which had been introduced by Senators Frist and Kennedy on November 15, 2001. S. 1765 incorporated ideas and objectives from several other Senate bioterrorism bills introduced in the wake of the anthrax attacks.[1] The Senate took up H.R. 3448 on December 20, 2001, following its passage in the House, substituted the text of S. 1765 and passed H.R. 3448, as amended, by unanimous consent. A conference report (H.Rept. 107-481) was filed on May 21, 2002. The next day the House agreed to the conference report by a vote of 425-1. The Senate approved the conference report 98-0 on May 23, 2002. The President signed H.R. 3448 into law (P.L. 107-188) on June 12, 2002.

Overview of P.L. 107-188

As enacted, P.L. 107-188 incorporates many of the provisions in the original House and Senate-passed bills. It adds to the programs and authorities established in Title III of the Public Health Service (PHS) Act by the Public Health Threats and Emergencies Act of 2000 (P.L. 106-505, Title I) and creates a new PHS Act Title XXVIII: National Preparedness for Bioterrorism and Other Public Health Emergencies. P.L. 107-188 is a 5-year authorization act, which calls for a total of $2.4 billion in funding for FY2002, $2.0 billion for FY2003, and such sums as may be necessary for the remaining years. The act authorizes grants to state and local health departments and hospitals to improve planning and preparedness activities, enhance laboratory capacity, and educate and train health care personnel. It also directs the

[1] Senate bioterrorism preparedness bills introduced in response to the September 11 attacks and the anthrax incidents include: the Biological and Chemical Weapons Preparedness Act of 2001 (S. 1486) introduced by Senator Edwards on October 3, 2001; the Biological and Chemical Attack Preparedness Act (S. 1508) introduced by Senator Corzine on October. 4, 2001; the State Bioterrorism Preparedness Act (S. 1520) introduced by Senator Bayh on October 9, 2001; the Protecting America's Children Against Terrorism Act (S. 1539) introduced by Senator Clinton on October 11, 2001; the Bioterrorism Awareness Act (S. 1548) introduced by Senator Carnahan on October 15, 2001; the Protecting the Food Supply from Bioterrorism Act (S. 1551) introduced by Senator Clinton on October 15, 2001; the Agricultural Bioterrorism Countermeasures Act of 2001 (S. 1563) introduced by Senator Hutchison on October 17, 2001; the Public Health Emergency Planning and Information Act of 2001 (S. 1574) introduced by Senator Rockefeller on October 25, 2001; the Pathogen Research, Emergency Preparedness and Response Efforts (PREPARE) Act of 2001 (S. 1635) introduced by Senator Hutchinson on November 6, 2001; and the Deadly Biological Agent Control Act of 2001 (S. 1661) introduced by Senator Feinstein on November 8, 2001.

Secretary to upgrade and renovate CDC's facilities. In addition, the act authorizes the HHS Secretary to purchase smallpox vaccine and expand the national stockpile of medicine and medical supplies to meet the nation's health security needs.

To help prevent bioterrorism and to establish a national database of potentially dangerous pathogens, P.L. 107-188 requires the HHS Secretary to register facilities and individuals in possession of biological agents and toxins that pose a severe threat to public health and safety, and to promulgate new safety and security requirements for such facilities and individuals. The act grants authority to the Secretary of Agriculture to establish a parallel set of requirements for facilities that handle agents and toxins that threaten crops and livestock. The bioterrorism legislation also incorporates language taken from S. 1275 that authorizes grants to states and localities to increase public access to defibrillators (i.e., devices that restore normal heart rhythm to patients in cardiac arrest by administering a controlled electric shock).

P.L. 107-188 contains several provisions to protect the nation's food and drug supply and enhance agricultural security. The act authorizes \$545 million for FDA and USDA to hire new border inspectors, develop new methods of detecting contaminated foods, work with state food safety regulators, and protect crops and livestock. It also provides FDA with new regulatory powers to require prior notice of all imported foods and detain suspicious foods for inspection. All foreign and domestic food facilities are required to register with the FDA. Finally, P.L. 107-188 includes a set of provisions aimed at protecting the nation's drinking water supply, including authorizing \$160 million to provide financial assistance to community water systems to conduct vulnerability assessments and prepare response plans.

The bioterrorism legislation also includes language reauthorizing the Prescription Drug User Fee Act (PDUFA), which was set to expire on September 30, 2002. Congress first enacted PDUFA in 1992.[2] The original law authorized the FDA to collect fees from pharmaceutical companies and use the funds to hire additional reviewers to expedite the drug review and approval process, in accordance with performance goals developed by the agency in consultation with the industry prior to PDUFA enactment. The 1992 law directed the FDA to provide Congress with an annual report on the agency's progress in achieving those goals. Encouraged by the success of the user fee program, Congress in 1997 reauthorized PDUFA through FY2002.[3] Under PDUFA II, the FDA tried to meet tighter performance goals, as well as achieve more transparency in the drug review process and better communication with drug makers and patient advocacy groups.

Table 1 below summarizes the bioterrorism legislation's authorizations of appropriations for FY2002 and FY2003. Only those authorizations that specify a dollar amount are included.

[2] P.L. 102-571, 21 U.S.C. Section 379(g).

[3] PDUFA reauthorization was included in Title I of the Food and Drug Administration Modernization Act of 1997, P.L. 105-115.

Table 1. P.L. 107-188: Authorizations of Appropriations for FY2002 and FY2003 ($ millions)

	FY2002	FY2003
Title I: National Preparedness for Bioterrorism and Other Public Health Emergencies		
Grants to state and local governments	No provision	$1,080
Grants for hospital preparedness	No provision	$520
Upgrading CDC	$300	$300
Strategic National Stockpile	$640	Such sums as may be necessary
Smallpox vaccine	$509	Such sums as may be necessary
Antimicrobial resistance	$25	$25
Emergency health professional verification system	$2	Such sums as may be necessary
Public access defibrillation programs	$5	$30
Dept. of Veterans Affairs emergency preparedness	$133	Such sums as may be necessary
Title IIIA: Food Supply Safety and Security	$130	Such sums as may be necessary
Title IIIC: Agricultural Security	$415	Such sums as may be necessary
Title IV: Drinking water Safety and Security	$210	Such sums as may be necessary
Title V: FDA Drug-Related Authorizations	No provision	$10
Total	**$2,369**	**$1,965**

Table 2, provides a detailed side-by-side comparison of the provisions of P.L. 107-188 with preexisting law, where applicable. All the PHS Act Title III provisions relating to public health emergencies that were established by P.L. 106-505 (i.e., Sections 319, 319A–319G) are included in the table, regardless of whether they are amended by the bioterrorism bill. Unless specifically noted otherwise, the term Secretary refers to the Secretary of HHS.

Table 2. Comparison of P.L. 107-188 with Preexisting Law

Topic	Preexisting Law	P.L. 107-188
National Preparedness for Bioterrorism and Other Public Health Emergencies		
National Preparedness Plan, reports to Congress	No statutory provisions.	Adds a new Title XXVIII (Section 2801) to the Public Health Service (PHS) Act that requires the Secretary, building on existing authority in PHS Act Section 319A, to develop and implement a national plan to prepare for and respond to bioterrorism and other public health emergencies. Establishes five national preparedness goals: (i) assist state and local governments in the event of bioterrorism or other public health emergencies; (ii) ensure that state and local governments have the capacity to detect and respond to such emergencies; (iii) develop and maintain countermeasures; (iv) ensure coordination and minimize duplication of federal, state, and local planning, preparedness, and response activities; and (v) enhance hospital and other health care facility readiness. Requires the Secretary to coordinate with the activities of state and local governments and develop outcome measures to evaluate progress in implementing the national plan and achieving its five goals. Requires the Secretary to report to Congress within 1 year, and biennially thereafter, on progress made towards meeting the national preparedness goals, including recommendations for new legislative authority to protect public health. Clarifies that the Act does not expand or limit any of the Secretary's preexisting authorities. Requires the Secretary to report to Congress within 1 year

Topic	Preexisting Law	P.L. 107-188
		on: (i) the findings and recommendations of the National Advisory Committee on Children and Terrorism and the EPIC Advisory Committee; (ii) the vulnerability of rural and medically underserved communities to bioterrorism; (iii) recommendations for new legislative authority to strengthen rural and medically underserved communities; and (iv) the need for and benefits of a private-sector, community-based rapid response corps of medical volunteers. Requires the Secretary to conduct a study of best practices in local emergency response and report to Congress within 180 days. [Section 101]
Establishing public health capacities	Public Health Service (PHS) Act Section 319A requires the Secretary, together with state and local health officials, to establish what capacities are needed for national, state, and local public health systems to be able to detect, diagnose, and contain outbreaks of infectious disease, drug-resistant pathogens, or acts of bioterrorism. Authorizes $4 million for FY2001, and such sums as may be necessary for FY2002–FY2006.	No provisions.
Assessing public health needs	PHS Act Section 319B authorizes grants to states and local public health departments to evaluate the extent to which they can achieve the capacities identified pursuant to Section 319A. Requires the Secretary to develop a national framework for the evaluations. Authorizes $45 million for FY2001, and such sums as may be necessary for FY2002–FY2003.	No provisions.

Topic	Preexisting Law	P.L. 107-188
Assistant Secretary for Public Health Emergency Preparedness	No statutory provisions.	Adds a new Section 2811(a) to the PHS Act authorizing the appointment of an Assistant Secretary for Public Health Emergency Preparedness to oversee the National Disaster Medical System (see below) and coordinate all HHS response activities related to bioterrorism and other public health emergencies and interface with other federal agencies and state and local entities. [Section 102(a)]
Public health emergencies	PHS Act Section 319 authorizes the Secretary to respond to public health emergencies, including diseases, disorders, or bioterrorist attacks, by supporting grants, contracts, and investigations. Establishes the Public Health Emergency Fund and authorizes such sums as may be necessary. Requires an annual report to Congress on expenditures from the Fund.	Requires the Secretary to notify Congress within 48 hours of declaring a public health emergency. Provides that public health emergencies expire by announcement of the Secretary or after 90 days, whichever comes first, and permits the Secretary to renew emergency declarations, subject to the same 90-day limitation. [Section 144] Allows the Secretary during a public health emergency to waive deadlines for the submission of data and reports by individuals or public or private entities pursuant to any law administered by the Secretary. Requires the Secretary to notify Congress of such an action and publish a notice in the *Federal Register*. [Section 141]
National Disaster Medical System (NDMS)	No statutory provisions. The NDMS was established in 1984 as a partnership of four federal agencies (HHS, FEMA, DOD, VA), state and local governments, and the private sector to provide medical assistance and hospitalization for mass casualties in the event of a natural or man-made disaster. It consists of more than 7,000 volunteer health professionals and support personnel organized into medical response teams. For more information,	Adds a new Section 2811(b) to the PHS Act providing statutory authorization for the NDMS, to be coordinated by HHS, FEMA, DOD, and the VA, in collaboration with states and other appropriate public or private entities. Requires the Secretary within 1 year, and periodically thereafter, to conduct exercises to test the capability and timeliness of the NDMS to mobilize and respond effectively to a bioterrorist attack or other public health emergency. Appoints activated NDMS volunteers as

Topic	Preexisting Law	P.L. 107-188
	go to [http://ndms.dhhs.gov/NDMS/ndms.html].	temporary federal employees. Establishes liability protections, compensation for work injuries, and employment and reemployment rights for NDMS volunteers. Authorizes such sums as may be necessary for FY2002–FY2006 for NDMS operations and for the Assistant Secretary for Public Health Emergency Preparedness. [Section 102(b)] Requires the VA Secretary, in consultation with the Secretaries of HHS and DOD and the FEMA Director, to establish a training program to facilitate the participation of VA medical center staff in the NDMS. [Section 154(e)]
Upgrading CDC, national public health communications and surveillance networks	PHS Act Section 319D authorizes funds for the construction and renovation of CDC facilities, and to support the agency's activities to combat threats to public health. Authorizes $180 million for FY2001, and such sums as may be necessary for FY2002–FY2010. Since FY1999, CDC has awarded grants to all 50 states and some metropolitan health departments to enhance state and local laboratory capacity and to help develop the Health Alert Network (NAH), a national electronic communications network connecting all the components of the public health community. For more information, go to [http://www.bt.cdc.gov].	Amends PHS Act Section 319D by recognizing CDC's essential role in defending against and combating bioterrorism and other public health emergencies. Provides CDC's Director with multi-year contracting authority for facility construction, renovation, and security. Requires the Secretary to improve CDC's preparedness and response capacities. Provides for the establishment of public health communications and surveillance networks and requires the Secretary, within 1 year and in cooperation with health care providers and state and local public health officials, to establish technical and reporting standards for such networks. Authorizes $300 million for FY2002 and for FY2003, and such sums as may be necessary for FY2004–FY2006, to upgrade CDC's facilities. Authorizes such sums as may be necessary for FY2002–FY2006 for improving CDC's

Topic	Preexisting Law	P.L. 107-188
		capacities and establishing national communications and surveillance networks. [Section 103]
Federal working groups and advisory committees	PHS Act Section 319F requires the Secretary to: (i) establish, with the Secretary of Defense, an interagency working group on bioterrorism preparedness, and (ii) establish, in collaboration with the Director of FEMA, the Attorney General, and the Secretary of Agriculture, an interagency working group to address the public health and medical consequences of a bioterrorist attack.	Amends PHS Act Section 319F by replacing the two existing working groups with a single interagency working group on the prevention, preparedness, and response to bioterrorism and other public health emergencies, to be established by the Secretary in coordination with the Attorney General, the Directors of FEMA and Central Intelligence, the Secretaries of Agriculture, Defense, Energy, Labor, and Veterans Affairs, the EPA Administrator, and with other federal officials, as appropriate. Requires the working group, or its subcommittees, to meet periodically for the purpose of consultation on, assisting in, and making recommendations on a range of specified topics related to preparedness for and response to bioterrorism and other public health emergencies (including research and development of countermeasures to treat, prevent, and identify exposure to biological agents). [Section 108] Amends PHS Act Section 319F as follows: (i) establishes the National Advisory Committee on Children and Terrorism, and the Emergency Public Information and Communications (EPIC) Advisory Committee (both of which sunset after 1 year); (ii) requires the Secretary to develop a strategy for effectively communicating information on bioterrorism and other public health emergencies; and (iii) recommends establishing a federal web site on bioterrorism with links to state and local

Topic	Preexisting Law	P.L. 107-188
		government sites. Requires the Secretary, in consultation with other federal agencies, to conduct a study of the ability of local public health entities to maintain communications during a bioterrorist attack or other public health emergency. [Sections 104]
Education and training of health care personnel	PHS Act Section 319F requires the Secretary to develop programs to educate health professionals in recognizing and caring for victims of bioterrorist attacks, and programs to train laboratory personnel in identifying bioweapons.	Amends PHS Act Section 319F by requiring the Secretary, in collaboration with the interagency working group and professional organizations, to award grants: (i) to develop education materials to teach health officials and other emergency personnel to identify potential bioweapons and other dangerous agents and to care for victims of public health emergencies, recognizing the special needs of children and other vulnerable populations; (ii) to develop education materials for community-wide planning to respond to bioterrorism or other public health emergencies; (iii) to develop materials for proficiency testing of lab and other public health personnel for the recognition and identification of potential bioweapons and other dangerous agents; and (iv) to provide for the dissemination and teaching of these materials. Authorizes the Secretary, in consultation with the Attorney General and the FEMA Director, to provide technical assistance for emergency response personnel training carried out by the Justice Department and FEMA. [Section 105]
National Pharmaceutical Stockpile (NPS)	No statutory provisions. The NPS, which was established and is managed by the CDC, includes pharmaceuticals, vaccines, and medical supplies that	Provides statutory authorization for a Strategic National Stockpile of drugs, vaccines, medical devices, and other supplies to meet the nation's health security needs in the

Topic	Preexisting Law	P.L. 107-188
	can be deployed anywhere in the country in response to a public health emergency. For more information, go to [http://www.cdc.gov/nceh/nps/default.htm].	event of a bioterrorist attack or other public health emergency. Requires the Secretary to manage the stockpile, in coordination with the VA Secretary, and ensure its physical security. Protects information on stockpile locations from disclosure under the Freedom of Information Act. Authorizes $640 million for FY2002, and such sums as may be necessary for FY2003–FY2006. [Section 121]
Grants to address national shortages of specific types of health professionals	No applicable provisions, although PHS Act Titles VII (Health Professionals Education) and VIII (Nursing Workforce Development) authorize federal support for training of health professionals for specific purposes.	Adds a new Section 319H to the PHS Act establishing a grant program to provide financial assistance for the education and training of individuals in any category of the health professions where there is a shortage that the Secretary determines should be alleviated to improve public health emergency readiness. Authorizes sums as may be necessary for FY2002–FY2006. [Section 106]
Health professional volunteers	No applicable provisions.	Adds a new Section 319I to the PHS Act requiring the Secretary to establish a electronic database for the advance registration of health professionals to verify their credentials, licenses, accreditations, and hospital privileges when they volunteer to respond during public health emergencies. Authorizes the Secretary to encourage states to permit out-of-state health professionals to provide health services during public health emergencies. Authorizes $2 million for FY2002, and such sums as may be necessary for FY2003–FY2006. [Section 107]
State public emergency announcements	The Stafford Act (42 U.S.C. 5121 et seq.) authorizes federal assistance when the President determines that	Amends Section 613(b) of the Stafford Act by requiring states to include a plan for providing a coordinated public

Topic	Preexisting Law	P.L. 107-188
	a natural or manmade disaster has overwhelmed state and local resources. Stafford assistance is administered by the Federal Emergency Management Agency (FEMA).	communications response in their submission for federal funds to help pay for state emergency preparedness personnel and administrative expenses. [Section 151]
Quarantine and inspection	PHS Act Section 361 authorizes the Surgeon General, in consultation with the Secretary, to develop quarantine, inspection, fumigation, sanitation, and pest extermination regulations to prevent the introduction, transmission, or spread of communicable diseases. Section 363 authorizes the development of regulations for the apprehension and examination of infected individuals in times of war.	Amends PHS Act Sections 361 and 363 by expanding the authority of the Secretary, in consultation with the Surgeon General, to issue a quarantine rule or a rule providing for the apprehension of individuals during wartime. Permits federal regulations under Sections 361 and 363, as amended, to preempt state laws that conflict with the exercise of such federal authority. [Section 142]
GAO Report	PHS Act Section 319F requires a GAO report to Congress, within 6 months, on federal bioterrorism-related activities, including research, preparedness, and response. [This report, GAO-01-915, was issued by GAO on September 28, 2001.]	Requires a new GAO report to Congress on federal bioterrorism-related activities, including research, preparedness, and response. [Section 157]
Occupational safety and health	Section 22 of the Occupational Safety and Health Act of 1970 (29 U.S.C. 671) created the National Institute for Occupational Safety and Health (NIOSH) as the federal agency responsible for conducting research and making recommendations for the prevention of work-related disease and injury. NIOSH is part of the CDC.	Requires the Secretary, acting through the Director of NIOSH, to expand research on bioterrorism threats and attacks in the workplace. [Section 153]
Department of Veterans Affairs	No statutory provisions.	Directs the VA Secretary to enhance the readiness of VA medical centers and research facilities to respond to a chemical or biological attack, based on the results of an evaluation of the security needs at these facilities.

Topic	Preexisting Law	P.L. 107-188
		Requires the VA Secretary to develop a centralized tracking system for pharmaceuticals and medical supplies and equipment throughout the VA health care system, and train VA health care personnel in emergency medical response. Authorizes $100 million for FY2002, and such sums as may be necessary for FY2003–FY2006. Requires the VA Secretary, in consultation with the HHS Secretary, the American Red Cross, and the interagency working group, to provide mental health counseling to individuals seeking care at a VA medical center following a bioterrorist attack or other public health emergency. Authorizes $33 million for FY2002, and such sums as may be necessary for FY2003–FY2006. [Section 154]
Supplies and services in lieu of federal grant funds	No applicable provisions.	Adds a new Section 319J to the PHS Act allowing the Secretary to provide supplies, equipment, or services instead of, or in conjunction with, grants awarded under Sections 319 through 319I, or Section 319K. [Section 110]
Psychological impact of trauma	PHS Act Section 582 authorizes the Secretary to award grants to study the psychological impact of trauma, in order to improve the treatment children and youth that suffer from psychiatric disorders as a result of witnessing or experiencing traumatic events. Authorizes $50 million for FY2001, and such sums as may be necessary for FY2002–FY2003.	Extends grant authority and authorizes such sums as may be necessary for FY2003–FY2006. [Section 155]
Public access to automated external defibrillators	PHS Act Section 247 requires the Secretary, in consultation with other federal agencies and appropriate public and private entities, to establish	Community Access to Emergency Defibrillation Act of 2002: Adds a new Section 312 to the PHS Act authorizing grants to develop and implement public

Topic	Preexisting Law	P.L. 107-188
	guidelines for placing automated external defibrillators (AEDs) in federal buildings, and to publish in the *Federal Register* recommendations for AED placement. PHS Act Section 248 establishes the conditions under which a person who uses or attempts to use an AED in a medical emergency is immune from civil liability for any resulting harm to the victim.	access defibrillation programs. Funds may be used to purchase AEDs, to provide training in AED usage, to provide information to community members about the public access defibrillation program, to provide information to local emergency medical services on AED placement, and to encourage private companies to purchase AEDs. Authorizes $25 million for FY2003, and such sums as may be necessary for FY2004–FY2006. Adds a new Section 313 to the PHS Act authorizing grants to develop and implement innovative, community-based public access defibrillation demonstration projects. Authorizes $5 million for each of FY2002–FY2006. [Section 159]
Medicare, Medicaid, and the State Children's Health Insurance Program (SCHIP)		
Emergency waivers	Medicare covers medically necessary acute care and follow-up services (hospital, short-term nursing home care, physician services, home health and a variety of outpatient services) for all persons age 65 and over, as well as certain disabled persons. Medicare beneficiaries may receive services through the traditional fee-for-service setting or may enroll in a Medicare managed care plan through the Medicare + Choice (M+C) program. Medicaid covers acute and long-term care services for low-income persons who are aged, blind, disabled, members of families with dependent children, and certain other pregnant women and children. The State Children's Health Insurance Program (SCHIP) covers uninsured	Authorizes the Secretary to temporarily waive conditions of participation and other certification requirements for any entity that furnishes health care items or services to Medicare, Medicaid, or SCHIP beneficiaries in an emergency area during a declared disaster or public health emergency. In addition, during such an emergency, authorizes the Secretary to waive: (i) participation, state licensing (as long as equivalent licensure from another state is held and there is no exclusion from practicing in that state or any state in the emergency area), and pre-approval requirements for physicians and other practitioners; (ii) sanctions for failing to meet requirements for emergency transfers between hospitals; (iii) sanctions for physician self-referral; and (iv)

Topic	Preexisting Law	P.L. 107-188
	children living in families with income above applicable Medicaid standards, typically up to or above 200% of the federal poverty level. In all three programs, providers must meet certain standards in order to participate and receive reimbursement for services rendered to program beneficiaries. For example, hospitals and other facilities must meet established conditions of participation, and laboratories must be certified under the Clinical Laboratories Improvement Act (CLIA). Physicians must be licensed to provide medical services in the state where medical care is rendered, and must follow established rules for obtaining prior approval to deliver certain types of services. Also, physicians must not refer patients to medical entities with which they have a financial relationship. Other statutory provisions require hospitals to fully stabilize patients receiving emergency care prior to transfer to another medical facility.	limitations on payments for health care and services furnished to individuals enrolled in M+C plans when services are provided outside the plan. To the extent possible, the Secretary shall ensure that M+C enrollees do not pay more than would have been required had they received care within their plan network. Requires the Secretary to provide Congress with certification and written notice at least 2 days prior to exercising this waiver authority. Provides for the waiver authority to continue for 60 days. Permits the Secretary to extend the waiver period. Requires the Secretary, within 1 year after the end of the emergency, to provide Congress with an evaluation of this approach and recommendations for improvements under this waiver authority. [Section 143]
Regulation of the Use, Possession, and Transfer of Potentially Dangerous Biological Agents and Toxins		
HHS regulation of biological agents and toxins that pose a threat to public health and safety	The 1996 Antiterrorism and Effective Death Penalty Act (P.L. 104-132, Section 511(d)-(g)) required the Secretary to: (i) establish a list of biological agents that may pose a severe threat to public health and safety; and (ii) establish safety procedures for transferring listed agents and toxins, including measures to protect public safety, prevent access by terrorists, and ensure the availability of bioagents for	Codifies and expands provisions of P.L. 104-132 in the PHS Act under a new Section 351A. Requires the Secretary to: (i) establish and, at least biennially, review and, if necessary, revise a list of biological agents and toxins that may pose a severe threat to public health and safety; (ii) establish safety procedures for transferring listed agents and toxins, including measures to protect public safety, prevent access by terrorists, and ensure the

Topic	Preexisting Law	P.L. 107-188
	research, education, and other legitimate purposes. The regulations issued pursuant to the Act (i.e., 42 C.F.R. 72.6) include: (i) a list of 36 agents and toxins; (ii) registration requirements for facilities transferring these agents; (iii) transfer requirements; (iv) verification procedures including audit and quality control; (v) agent disposal requirements; and (vi) research and clinical exemptions.	availability of agents and toxins for research, education, and other legitimate purposes; (iii) establish standards and procedures for the possession and use of listed agents and toxins, including the same measures listed in (ii); (iv) require registration for the possession, use, and transfer of listed agents and toxins; and (v) maintain a national database of registered facilities and the location of listed agents and toxins. Directs the Secretary, in consultation with the Attorney General, to establish appropriate safety and security requirements for registered entities and individuals, commensurate with the level of risk to public health and safety. These requirements must ensure that persons registering facilities: (i) limit access to listed agents and toxins to only those individuals (employees) with a legitimate need; (ii) identify such individuals to the Secretary and the Attorney General for background screening; (iii) deny access to individuals determined by the Attorney General to be "restricted individuals" (see Criminal Penalties below); and (iv) limit or deny access to individuals found to meet other specified criteria. Requires prompt screening and notification by the Attorney General and Secretary and provides for an expedited screening process where the registered person has demonstrated good cause. Establishes procedures for the review of denials based on the screening process. Requires persons seeking to register a facility, as well as individuals seeking to register themselves, to be screened

Topic	Preexisting Law	P.L. 107-188
		in the same manner as individuals working at a registered facility, but without the option of expedited review. Allows the Secretary to exempt federal, state, and local government facilities from screening. Requires that the Secretary be promptly notified of the theft or loss of listed agents or toxins. Authorizes the Secretary to conduct compliance inspections. Exempts from the above requirements clinical and diagnostic labs presented with a listed agent or toxin for diagnosis, verification, or proficiency testing, provided that they report the identification of the agent or toxin to the Secretary and transfer or destroy it. Exempts agents or toxins licensed or approved under specified federal laws, unless the Secretary determines that additional regulation is necessary to protect public health and safety. Permits the Secretary to exempt investigational products being used in research or clinical trials and requires the Secretary to make a prompt (within 14 days) determination on a request for such an exemption. Permits the Secretary to grant temporary exemptions during public health and agricultural emergencies. Protects information collected under the above requirements for the possession, use, and transfer of listed agents and toxins from disclosure under the Freedom of Information Act. Establishes civil penalties of up to $500,000 for violations of Section 351A. Requires prompt notification of the Secretary in the event of an unintentional release of a listed agent or toxin. Requires

Topic	Preexisting Law	P.L. 107-188
		the Secretary to report to Congress within 1 year. Authorizes such sums as may be necessary for FY2002–FY2007. [Section 201]
Implementation time frame for HHS regulations	No statutory provisions.	Requires that all persons in possession of listed agents or toxins notify the Secretary within 90 days, based on guidance issued by the Secretary within 30 days. Requires the Secretary within 180 days to issue an interim final rule for carrying out Section 351A (including time frames for the applicability of the rule to minimize disruption of research and education). [Section 202] Repeals current law (i.e., P.L. 104-132, Section 511(d)-(g)). [Section 204]
USDA regulation of biological agents and toxins that pose a threat to agriculture	No statutory provisions.	Gives USDA comparable regulatory authority to that provided to HHS under Section 201 of the Act for regulating the use, possession, and transfer of listed biological agents and toxins that may pose a severe threat to animal or plant health, or to animal or plant products. The USDA provisions differ from those of HHS in the criteria used to develop a list of agriculturally significant biological agents and toxins. Also, there is no mandated denial of access for "restricted individuals" because possession of USDA-listed agents by such persons is not a federal crime. Additional provisions address overlap agents and toxins that appear in both the HHS and the USDA list. [Section 212]
Implementation time frame for USDA regulations	No statutory provisions.	Requires the USDA Secretary to issue an interim final rule establishing the initial list of agents and toxins within 60 days and, no later than 60 days after that date, requires

Topic	Preexisting Law	P.L. 107-188
		all persons in possession of listed agents or toxins to notify the Secretary. Requires the USDA Secretary within 180 days to issue an interim final rule for carrying out Section 212 of the Act (including time frames for the applicability of the rule to minimize disruption of research and education). [Section 213]
HHS-USDA coordination	No statutory provisions.	Requires the Secretaries of HHS and Agriculture to coordinate activities regarding overlap agents and toxins that appear in both lists, so as to minimize the administrative burden on those persons subject to both sets of regulations. Requires both Secretaries, within 180 days, to enter into a memorandum of understanding providing for the development of a single system of registration for persons who use, possess, or transfer overlap agents or toxins, and to coordinate inspections and enforcement. Requires the Secretaries to issue joint regulations for the use, possession, and transfer of overlap agents and toxins within 18 months. [Section 221]
Criminal penalties	Section 175 of the U.S. Criminal Code (i.e., 18 U.S.C. 175): (i) prohibits the production, stockpiling, transfer, acquisition, or possession of biological agents for use as a weapon, subject to fines and/or imprisonment for life or any term of years; and (ii) establishes fines and/or up to 10 years imprisonment for individuals who knowingly possess any biological agent, toxin, or delivery system of a type and in a quantity not reasonably justified by research or other peaceful purposes. Section 175b prohibits "restricted	Amends 18 U.S.C. 175b by adding the following criminal penalties: (i) fines and/or up to 5 years imprisonment for anyone who transfers a listed agent or toxin to a person whom the transferor knows or has reasonable cause to believe has not obtained a registration; and (ii) fines and/or up to 5 years imprisonment for unregistered persons in possession of listed agents or toxins. Note: These new penalties apply to both the HHS and USDA regulations described above. [Section 231]

Topic	Preexisting Law	P.L. 107-188
	individuals" (i.e., indicted criminals, illegal aliens, and other specified individuals) from possessing, shipping, or receiving listed agents or toxins, subject to fines and/or up to 10 years imprisonment. Section 176 provides for the seizure, forfeiture, and destruction of biological weapons.	
State and Local Preparedness and Response Capacity		
Core capacity grants to state and local public health agencies	PHS Act Section 319C authorizes grants to states and local governments, after they have completed a Section 319B evaluation, to address core public health capacity needs. Requires the Secretary to report to Congress on activities carried out under Sections 319A, 319B, and 319C by January 1, 2005. Authorizes $50 million for FY2001, and such sums as may be necessary for FY2002–FY2006.	Deletes PHS Act Section 319C(f) (i.e., Authorization of Appropriations). [Section 131(b)]
Bioterrorism preparedness grants to states and local public health agencies, and health care facilities	PHS Act Section 319F(c) authorizes grants to states, localities, and health care facilities to increase their capacity to detect, diagnose, and respond to bioterrorist attacks, including training of personnel. [Note: For all activities under Section 319F, authorizes $215 million for FY2001, and such sums as may be necessary for FY2002–FY2006.]	Adds a new Section 319C-1 to the PHS Act authorizing grants to states and local governments to improve preparedness and response to bioterrorism and other public health emergencies. Eligible entities must have completed a Section 319B evaluation of core public health capacity needs and must, within 60 days of receiving an award, submit an emergency preparedness and response plan (including performance measures) describing the activities to be carried out by the entity to address identified needs. Use of funds for preparedness and response to bioterrorism and outbreaks of infectious disease takes priority over other public health emergencies, subject to any modification in the

Topic	Preexisting Law	P.L. 107-188
		assessment of risk by the Secretary. Authorizes $1.6 billion for FY2003: $1.08 billion for block grants to states and territories based on population, with each state/territory guaranteed a minimum level of funding; and $520 million for grants to states for hospital preparedness. Authorizes such sums as may be necessary for FY2004–FY2006. Note: The requirement that public health preparedness funding be awarded as block grants applies only to FY2003; greater flexibility in awarding funding is provided to the Secretary beyond FY2003. [Section 131(a)]
Grants to hospitals	No applicable provisions.	Adds a new Section 319C-2 to the PHS Act authorizing grants to improve community and hospital preparedness for bioterrorism and other public health emergencies. Eligible entities must be a partnership between one or more hospitals (or other health care facilities) and one or more states and/or local governments. Grant proposals must be coordinated and consistent with the state's emergency preparedness and response plan. Use of funds for preparedness and response to bioterrorism and outbreaks of infectious disease takes priority over other public health emergencies, subject to any modification in the assessment of risk by the Secretary. Authorizes such sums as may be necessary for FY2004–FY2006. [Section 131(a)]
Demonstration grants	PHS Act Section 319G authorizes up to three demonstration grants for up to 5 years to states, localities, or non-profit organizations to carry out	No provisions.

Topic	Preexisting Law	P.L. 107-188
	programs to improve biopathogen detection, develop plans for responding to bioterrorist attacks, and train response personnel. Requires a GAO report to Congress at the conclusion of the demonstration programs describing the capabilities of the grantees. Authorizes $6 million for FY2001, and such sums as may be necessary for FY2002–FY2006.	
Countermeasures (Research, Development, and Production of New Vaccines, Drugs, and Technologies)		
Smallpox vaccine	No statutory provisions. Existing supplies of smallpox vaccine consist of 15.4 million doses of freeze-dried vaccine (produced by Wyeth Laboratories) that HHS indicates could be expanded to 77 million doses by 1:5 dilution, plus another 75–90 million doses of a different vaccine (produced by Aventis Pasteur) that HHS is testing for safety and effectiveness. In addition, HHS has contracted with Acambis Inc. to produce a total of 209 million doses of a new type of smallpox vaccine by the end of 2002 (the new vaccine needs FDA approval before it can be used).	Requires the Secretary to ensure that the national stockpile contains enough smallpox vaccine to meet the nation's health security needs. Authorizes $509 million for FY2002, and such sums as may be necessary for FY2003–FY2006, to purchase smallpox vaccine. [Section 121]
FDA approval of drugs and biologics	Under the Federal Food, Drug, and Cosmetic Act (FFDCA; 21 U.S.C. 301 et seq.), manufacturers of drugs and biologics (e.g., vaccines) must provide clinical trial data to demonstrate that their product is safe and effective, in order to obtain FDA marketing approval. The FFDCA provides for the designation of products as fast track to expedite the approval process.	Authorizes the Secretary to designate a priority countermeasure as a fast-track product for accelerated approval by the FDA. Permits a drug for which FDA approval is being sought on the basis of animal data to be designated a fast-track product. Requires the FDA, within 90 days, to issue as a final rule the October 5, 1999 proposed rule (64 *Fed. Reg.* 53960) permitting the use of animal data for demonstrating the effectiveness of new

Topic	Preexisting Law	P.L. 107-188
		drugs and vaccines when ethical issues preclude conducting human clinical trials. (Note: FDA published a final rule on May 31, 2002 (67 *Fed. Reg.* 37988).) [Section 122, 123]
Security at research and production facilities	No applicable provisions.	Adds a new Section 319K to the PHS Act authorizing the Secretary, in consultation with the Secretary of Defense and the Attorney General, to provide technical or other assistance to enhance security at facilities that develop, produce, distribute, or store priority countermeasures. [Section 124]
Research and development	PHS Act Section 319F requires the Secretary, in consultation with the interagency working group, to conduct research on the epidemiology and pathogenesis of biopathogens, diagnostic tests for biopathogens, and vaccines and other therapeutics.	Directs the Secretary to accelerate research and development on priority pathogens (as determined by the NIH Director in consultation with the interagency working group) and priority countermeasures. Requires the Secretary to consider research collaboration with the VA. Defines priority countermeasures as any drug, vaccine, biological product, device, or diagnostic test that the Secretary determines to be a priority to treat, identify, or prevent infection by a listed biological agent or toxin, or harm from any other agent that may cause a public health emergency. [Section 125]
Detection, identification, diagnosis, and surveillance technologies	No applicable provisions.	Requires the Secretary of Energy and the Administrator of the National Nuclear Safety Administration, in coordination with the interagency working group, to expand research on the rapid detection and identification of biopathogens and other agents that may cause a public health emergency, and report to Congress within 180 days. Authorizes such sums as may be necessary for

Topic	Preexisting Law	P.L. 107-188
		FY2002–FY2006. [Section 152] Requires the Secretary, in consultation with the interagency working group, to evaluate new and emerging technologies for improving surveillance of public health emergencies and report to Congress within 180 days, and periodically thereafter. [Section 126]
Potassium iodide	Under general authority provided by the Atomic Energy Act of 1954 (42 U.S.C. 2011 et seq.) and the Energy Reorganization Act of 1974 (42 U.S.C. 5801 et seq.), the Nuclear Regulatory Commission (NRC) requires that the use of potassium iodide (KI) by the public be considered during development of nuclear power plant emergency plans (see 10 C.F.R. 50.47). Under a policy adopted December 22, 2000, NRC will pay for state KI stockpiles. Note: Taking KI in the event of a nuclear attack or accident slows a person's uptake of radioactive iodine by flooding the thyroid gland with nonradioactive iodine.	Directs the President to provide KI from the national stockpile to state and local governments that submit a plan for the local stockpiling and distribution to everyone within 20 miles of a nuclear power plant. Additional eligibility requirements apply to local government plans. Requires the President within 1 year, in consultation with appropriate federal, state, and local agencies, to establish guidelines on stockpiling, distributing, and using KI in the event of a nuclear incident. Requires the President within 6 months to report to Congress on state and local KI stockpiles. Directs the President to request a study by the National Academy of Sciences on the safest and most effective way to distribute and administer KI on a large scale, to be submitted to Congress within 6 months. Permits the program to be terminated if the President determines that there are more effective measures to protect against thyroid disease. [Section 127]
Antimicrobial Resistance		
Combating antimicrobial resistance	PHS Act 319E requires the Secretary to establish an Antimicrobial Resistance Task Force to coordinate federal programs on antimicrobial resistance and to work on surveillance plans and information systems	Amends PHS Act Section 319E to authorize additional research on priority pathogens. Authorizes $25 million for FY2002 and for FY2003, and such sums as may be necessary for FY2004–FY2006. [Section 109]

Topic	Preexisting Law	P.L. 107-188
	for detection and control of drug-resistant pathogens. Authorizes research and development initiatives for new antimicrobial drugs and diagnostics. Directs the Secretary to conduct a nationwide campaign to educate the public and health care professionals about the appropriate use of antibiotics. Authorizes grants for public health agencies to combat antimicrobial resistance. Authorizes demonstration grants for hospitals, clinics, and other entities to promote the judicious use of antibiotics and to control the spread of resistant infections. Authorizes $40 million for FY2001, and such sums as may be necessary for FY2002–FY2006.	
Drug and Device Supply Safety and Security		
Drug and device importation	FFDCA Section 510(i) requires foreign drug and device manufacturers that import into the United States to register with the Secretary their name, place of business, and the name of their U.S. agent. Section 801 governs the import and export of food, drugs, devices, and other items, and specifies the circumstances under which imported articles are inspected, detained, or refused entry into the United States.	Amends Section 510(i) of the FFDCA by requiring annual registration, through electronic means, of foreign manufacturers importing drugs and devices into the United States. Requires the registration to include the name of each importer and agent used by the manufacturer, and the name of each person who imports or offers for import such drugs or devices. Amends Section 801 by refusing entry to drugs or devices that are offered for importation, if the import declaration does not include registration information about the manufacturer. Requires refused articles to be held at the port of entry or removed to a secure facility, as appropriate, until registration information is provided. [Section 321]

Topic	Preexisting Law	P.L. 107-188
Import components intended for export	FFDCA Section 301 is the prohibited acts and penalties section of the statute. Section 801 governs the import and export of food, drugs, devices, and other items, and specifies the circumstances under which imported articles are inspected, detained, or refused entry into the United States.	Amends Section 801 of the FFDCA mandating a chain-of-possession identification and a customs bond for firms seeking to import components of drugs, devices, food additives, color additives, or dietary supplements for further processing and export. Requires certificates of analysis to identify such components, except for components of devices and blood and tissue components. Permits the Secretary to exclude from importation any article for which there is credible evidence or information indicating that the article is not intended to be imported for export. Amends Section 301 making it illegal to knowingly submit false statements, certificates, records, or reports required under Section 801, as amended. [Section 322]
Additional Authorizations of Appropriations for FDA Drug Regulation		
Drug safety	The Office of Drug Safety in FDA's Center for Drug Evaluation and Research (CDER) conducts postmarket surveillance and monitors adverse drug reactions and medication errors.	Authorizes the following amounts for the Office of Drug Safety (ODS): FY2003=ODS FY2002 appropriation + $5 million; FY2004=ODS FY2002 appropriation + $10 million; each subsequent fiscal year=ODS FY2004 appropriation adjusted for inflation since beginning of FY2004. [Section 521]
Drug marketing, advertising, and communications	FDA/CDER's Division of Drug Marketing, Advertising, and Communications is responsible for ensuring that prescription drug information provided by manufacturers is truthful, balanced, and accurate.	Authorizes the following amounts for the Division of Drug Marketing, Advertising, and Communications, expressed as an increase over its FY2002 appropriation: FY2003=$2.5 million; FY2004=$4 million; FY2005=$5.5 million; FY2006=$7.5 million; FY2007=$7.5 million. [Section 522]

Topic	Preexisting Law	P.L. 107-188
Generic drugs	FDA/CDER's Office of Generic Drugs is responsible for reviewing and approving generic product applications.	Authorizes the following amounts for the Office of Generic Drugs, expressed as an increase over its FY2002 appropriation: FY2003=$3 million; FY2004=$6 million; FY2005=$9 million; FY2006=$12 million; FY2007=$15 million. [Section 523]
Food Supply Safety and Security		
Food safety and security strategy.	Executive Order 13100 created the President's Council on Food Safety, headed by the Secretaries of Agriculture and HHS, the EPA Administrator, and the Assistant to the President for Science and Technology. On January 18, 2001, the Council published a strategic plan for food safety, which contained recommendations on making statutory changes to unify federal food safety regulations.	Requires the Council, in consultation with the Secretaries of Transportation and Treasury, other interested federal agencies, states, the food industry, scientific organizations, and consumer and producer groups to develop a crisis communications and education strategy against bioterrorist threats to the food supply. Requires the strategic plan to address threat assessments, technologies and procedures for securing food processing facilities, modes of transportation of foods, response and notification procedures, and public risk communication plans. Authorizes $750,000 for FY2002, and such sums as may be necessary in each subsequent fiscal year, to implement the strategy. [Section 301]
Protection against adulteration of food.	FFDCA Chapter IV prohibits the entry into interstate commerce of adulterated or misbranded foods. FDA monitors through inspections whether food manufacturers adhere to their legal responsibility to produce food that is not defective, unsafe, filthy, or produced under unsanitary conditions. FFDCA Section 801 gives general authority to the Secretary to sample and regulate imported products.	Amends FFDCA Section 801 to create a new subsection (h): to authorize the Secretary to increase inspections for the detection of intentional adulteration of imported food; to give high priority to improving FDA's food import information management systems; to improve linkages with other federal regulatory agencies, states and Indian tribes (under the Indian Self-Determination and Education Assistance Act) that share responsibility for food safety; to fund research on improved testing and

Topic	Preexisting Law	P.L. 107-188
		sampling methods to rapidly detect intentionally adulterated food at ports of entry; to coordinate with the heads of CDC, NIH, EPA and USDA on the research; and to provide an annual report to Congress on the research findings. Requires the Secretary, acting through FDA and not later than 6 months after enactment, to complete an assessment of threats to food posed by intentional adulteration and report to Congress. Authorizes a total of $100 million for FY2002, and such sums as are necessary for FY2003–FY2006, to carry out these activities. [Section 302]
Administrative detention	FFDCA Section 304 allows for the seizure of food in interstate commerce under restricted circumstances. FFDCA Section 301 lists prohibited acts; Section 801 is the general authority for regulating imports and exports.	Amends FFDCA Section 304 to add a new subsection (h) to authorize the detention of food for 20 days, and if needed for 30 days and to institute an action if an officer or qualified employee of FDA has credible evidence (and the Secretary or Secretary's designee approves) showing the food presents a threat of serious adverse health consequences or death to humans or animals, with expedited procedures for perishable foods. A detained food may be placed in a secure facility, may be marked or labeled as detained, and cannot be transferred out of detention unless it is released by the Secretary or the detention period expires, whichever occurs first. The person responsible for the detained food can appeal the decision to the Secretary. After an appeal is filed, within 5 days the Secretary must provide for an informal hearing to confirm or end the detention order. If the Secretary fails to act, the detention is terminated. An appeal is also

Topic	Preexisting Law	P.L. 107-188
		terminated if the district court files an injunction or restraining order on the food. Amends FFDCA Section 301 prohibiting the removal of a detained product or any mark or label identifying the product as detained. Amends FFDCA Section 801 to authorize an FDA officer or qualified employee to request the Treasury Secretary to temporarily hold imported food at a port for 24 hours, if FDA has credible evidence indicating that the food presents a threat of serious adverse health consequences or death to humans or animals, and the FDA official is unable to inspect, examine, or investigate the import to determine whether to detain the food. If necessary, the Treasury Secretary may remove the food to a secure facility from where it will not be delivered pursuant to the execution of a bond. Requires that the Secretary notify the state in which the involved port is located. [Section 303]
Debarment for repeated or serious food import violations.	FFDCA Section 306 gives the Secretary authority to debar, temporarily deny approval, or suspend the rights of individuals who have been convicted of a felony to submit an application for approval of a drug.	Amends FFDCA Section 306 to debar from importing foods any person who is convicted of a felony related to the importation of food or who repeatedly imports, or knows, or should have known, that the imported food was adulterated. Requires food imported by a debarred person to be refused admission and held in a secure facility, as appropriate, unless a non-debarred person establishes that the food complies with the requirements of the FFDCA, as determined by the Secretary. Imported food that is refused admission may not be delivered pursuant to the execution of a bond under Section 801(b). Amends

Topic	Preexisting Law	P.L. 107-188
		FFDCA Section 301 prohibiting the importing of a food by a debarred person. Amends FFDCA Section 801 to include in the definition of "adulterated food" any food imported by debarred persons as a prohibited act under Section 301. The prohibited act is not intended to include an innocent purchaser who did not know of the importer's debarred status. Authorizes the Secretary to terminate the debarment of companies or persons. [Section 304]
Registration of food facilities.	Currently, only states have records of food processing, packing and holding facilities. The federal government must ask the states for this information.	Creates a new Section 415 in the FFDCA requiring all facilities, domestic and foreign, that manufacture, process, and handle food to register with the Secretary on a one-time basis and give timely updates of all the identities (trade names) under which business is conducted, names and addresses of the facilities, and general food categories (as identified in 21 C.F.R. 170.3). Foreign registrants must name a U.S. agent. Requires the Secretary to give each facility a number and the failure of a facility to register is a prohibited act under FFDCA Section 301. Protect the list of registrants from disclosure under the Freedom of Information Act. Exempts restaurants, certain retail stores, nonprofit food establishments, fishing vessels, and farms from registration requirements. Registration does not imply a license. Amends 801 to prohibit foods from being imported from unregistered foreign facilities. Adds that the Secretary may provide for and encourage the use of electronic submissions to register as long as there are authorization protocols used to identify the registrant and

Topic	Preexisting Law	P.L. 107-188
		validate the data. Requires the Secretary within 18 months to promulgate regulations for facilities to register. If the final regulations had not become effective after 18 months, the requirements for registration will be self-executing. [Section 305]
Maintenance and inspection of records for foods	FDCA Section 701(a) authorizes FDA to promulgate regulations to enforce the Act. FFDCA Section 704 authorizes FDA to conduct factory inspections. Currently, FDA inspectors have access to company records but can only request access to copy, and verify records for restricted medical devices, prescription drugs, not for foods. Inspectors may not require that records be kept nor do officials have authority to copy records found during inspections.	Adds a new Section 414 to the FFDCA allowing the Secretary to inspect records, if a food is believed to be adulterated and presents a threat of serious adverse health consequences or death to humans or animals. Inspectors must present credentials and written notice in a reasonable manner to access and copy all records related to the food to help the Secretary decide if the food is a threat to health. Excludes restaurants and farms. The Secretary is to consider the size of a business in promulgating regulations. Requires records by persons who manufacture, process, pack, transport, distribute, receive, hold, or import food to be kept no longer than 2 years. The Secretary will use the records to identify the immediate previous sources and immediate subsequent recipients of food. including its packaging. Excludes records on USDA-regulated foods (meat, poultry, and egg products). Requires procedures to protect trade secrets or confidential information. Inspection of records does not extend to recipes for food, or financial, pricing, personnel, research, or sales data (other than shipment data regarding sales). Amends FFDCA Section 704(a) to add a clause to allow the inspection of all records and other information described in the new Section 414.

Topic	Preexisting Law	P.L. 107-188
		Requires final record keeping rules to be issued within 18 months. [Section 306]
Prior notice of imported food shipments	Under FFDCA Section 801, a food that (i) is found to be manufactured, processed, or packed under unsanitary conditions, (ii) is forbidden or restricted in the producing country or from where it was exported, or (iii) is adulterated or misbranded at the border, can have its admission deferred while the food is reconditioned, relabeled or destroyed.	Adds a new section 801(m)(1) to the FFDCA to require the Secretary, after consultation with the Secretary of the Treasury, to promulgate regulations, not later than 18 months after enactment, requiring that the importer give notice that a food will be presented for import. Requires that the notice include the following: a description of the food; the identity of the manufacturer and shipper and, if possible, the grower; the country of origin of the food; the country from which the article is shipped; and the anticipated U.S. port of entry. Requires the Secretary to establish by regulation the period of time for prior notice, that must be no less than the minimum amount of time necessary for the Secretary to receive, review, and respond to the notice, but that may not exceed 5 days. In developing these regulations, the Secretary should consider the effect on commerce, locations of U.S. ports, the transport modes, the types of food, and other such considerations. Requires that food without a notice be held at the port of entry until such notice is delivered to the Secretary and found to be in order. Food so held may not be delivered pursuant to the execution of a bond under Section 801(b) and may be taken to a secure facility, as appropriate. During this period, the Secretary will decide if there is evidence or information on whether the food presents a threat to health. All USDA-regulated foods (i.e., meat, poultry, and egg products) are exempt

Topic	Preexisting Law	P.L. 107-188
		from this section. Amends Section 301 prohibiting imports of food without prior notice. If the final rules are not effective within 18 months, the requirement for an import notice is self executing and will take effect so that notice must be given not less than 8 hours nor more than 5 days when a food is be offered for import. [Section 307]
Authority to mark articles refused admission into the United States.	FFDCA Section 403 defines misbranded foods as food whose labeling or advertising is false or misleading. Section 801(a) gives the Secretary the general authority to refuse imports deemed adulterated or misbranded.	Amends Sections 403 and 801(a) definitions of misbranded food to include food that has been refused admission to the United States and not destroyed, and which presents a threat of serious adverse health consequences or death, unless the packaging is clearly and conspicuously labeled *United States: Refused Entry* at the expense of the food's owner until the food is brought into compliance. If there is an adverse health threat, the Secretary must notify the owner or consignee that the food presents a threat. Nothing in this section limits the Secretaries of HHS or Treasury to require marketing the refused articles under any other provision of law. [Section 308]
Prohibition against port shopping	FFDCA Section 402 defines "adulterated" food as any food that bears or contains any poisonous or deleterious substance which may render it injurious to health.	Amends FFDCA Section 402 to require that an importer offering food that has been refused admission prove at his own expense that the food is in compliance with the applicable requirements of the Act. [Section 309]
Notices to states regarding imported food	No statutory provisions.	Amends Chapter IX of the FFDCA to add a new Section 908 to require that the Secretary notify the states that hold or will hold imported food, and the states where the manufacturer, packer, or distributor of the imported food is located, when there is credible evidence that it presents

Topic	Preexisting Law	P.L. 107-188
		a threat of serious adverse health consequences or death to humans or animals. Requires the Secretary to request that states take appropriate action to protect the public health. [Section 310]
Grants to states for inspections	FFDCA Section 702 states that the Secretary is authorized to conduct food inspections (examinations and investigations) through officers and employees of HHS, or any health, food, or drug officer of a state that has been duly commissioned by the Secretary as an officer of the Department.	Amends Chapter IX of the FFDCA to add a new Section 909 authorizing the Secretary to make grant to states for increased food safety inspection, examinations, and investigations under Section 702, and to cover the costs of taking appropriate actions to protect the public health as required under Section 908. Authorizes $10 million for FY2002, and such sums as may be necessary for FY2003–FY2006. [Section 311]
Surveillance and information grants and authorities	FoodNet, established in 1995 by USDA and FDA, tracks the incidence of illnesses caused by nine pathogens in nine geographic areas across the United States. PulseNet compares genetic patterns of bacteria isolated from patients with foodborne illness and/or contaminated food.	Amends PHS Act Title III, Part B to create a new Section 317R to authorize $19.5 million for FY2002, and such sums as may be necessary for FY2003–FY2006, in grants to states, and Indian tribes to expand the number participating in FoodNet and PulseNet and other surveillance networks and to maintain technical and laboratory capacity needed for such participation. [Section 312]
Surveillance of zoonotic diseases.	CDC has more than 20 surveillance programs that monitor outbreaks of food borne illness caused by specific pathogens.	Requires the Secretary to coordinate surveillance of zoonotic diseases (i.e., animal diseases communicable to man) through FDA, CDC, and USDA. [Section 313]
Authority to commission other federal officials to conduct inspections.	FFDCA Section 702 states that the Secretary is authorized to conduct food inspections (examinations and investigations) through officers and employees of HHS, or any health, food, or drug officer of a state that has been duly commissioned by the Secretary as	Amends FFDCA Section 702 to authorize the Secretary to commission other federal officials to conduct inspections, examinations, and investigations, pursuant to a memorandum of understanding (MOU) between the Secretary and the head of the agency to which the other

Topic	Preexisting Law	P.L. 107-188
	an officer of the Department.	officials belong. Inspections can take place only at facilities or other locations that are jointly regulated by HHS and the other agency. Requires the Secretary and the other agency head to report to Congress on the number of persons that carried out activities under the MOU, and the number of additional investigations and foods inspected or examined as a result of the MOU. [Section 314]
Rule of construction.	USDA regulates meat under the Federal Meat Inspection Act (21 U.S.C. 601 et seq.), poultry under the Poultry Products Inspection Act (21 U.S.C. 451 et seq.), and processed egg products under the Egg Products Inspection Act (21 U.S.C. 1031 et seq.).	Prohibits FDA from regulating any food under USDA's jurisdiction. [Section 315]
Agricultural Security		
USDA activities	USDA's Food Safety and Inspection Service (FSIS) inspects meat, poultry, and processed egg products sold for human consumption for safety, wholesomeness, and proper labeling. The Animal and Plant Inspection Service (APHIS) inspects cargo and passengers at U.S. ports for animal and plant pests, quarantines some of these products, and responds to animal disease outbreaks. The Agricultural Research Service (ARS) conducts research on animal diseases and food safety to support other USDA regulatory responsibilities.	Authorizes $15 million for FY2002, and such sums as may be necessary for each subsequent fiscal year, for enhanced FSIS inspections domestically and internationally and collaboration with other federal agencies. Authorizes $30 million for FY2002, and such sums as may be necessary for each subsequent fiscal year, for APHIS for increased inspections, cooperative agreements with state and private veterinarians, and an automated, integrated, interagency emergency warning, response, and record-keeping system. Authorizes $180 million for FY2002, and such sums as may be necessary for FY2003–FY2006, to upgrade biosecurity at ARS labs in New York and Iowa. Authorizes the appropriation of such sums as necessary for: (i) grants not exceeding $50,000 to land grant colleges of agriculture for

Topic	Preexisting Law	P.L. 107-188
		reviewing security standards and practices; and (ii) grants not exceeding $100,000 to agricultural producer groups to develop and implement on-farm biosecurity education programs. Authorizes $190 million for FY2002, and such sums as may be necessary in subsequent years, to support ARS and federal-state cooperative research on bioterrorism prevention, preparedness, and response; to strengthen coordination with U.S. intelligence agencies; and to develop an early warning surveillance system for agricultural bioterrorism. Establishes civil fines and criminal penalties for acts of terrorism against animal enterprises. [Sections 331–336]
Drinking Water Security and Safety		
Vulnerability assessments and emergency response plans	PHS Act Title XIV, the Safe Drinking Water Act (SDWA), authorizes federal regulation of public water systems, particularly through a program that regulates contaminants in public water supplies. The Act defines a community water system as a public water system that serves at least 15 service connections used by year-round residents or that regularly serves at least 25 year-round residents. The SDWA is administered and enforced by the Environmental Protection Agency (EPA).	Adds a new Section 1433 to the SDWA to require each community water system serving 3,300 or more individuals to conduct a vulnerability assessment. Requires EPA, not later than August 1, 2002, to provide information to these systems concerning probable threats. Establishes deadlines for community water systems to certify to EPA that they have conducted vulnerability assessments and to submit to EPA a copy of the assessment. Certifications and submissions must be made before March 31, 2003, by systems serving 100,000+ persons; December 31, 2003, by systems serving 50,000–99,999 persons; and June 30, 2004, by systems serving 3,300–49,999 persons. Exempts assessments from disclosure under the Freedom of Information Act and requires EPA to develop protocols to protect the

Topic	Preexisting Law	P.L. 107-188
		assessments from unauthorized disclosure. Provides that any individual designated by the Administrator who acquires assessments or information from them and who knowingly or recklessly reveals such information to unauthorized individuals shall be subject to up to 1 year imprisonment or a fine, unless the information is revealed for specified purposes. Requires each community water system serving 3,300+ individuals to prepare or revise an emergency response plan incorporating the results of the vulnerability assessment. Systems must certify to EPA, within 6 months of completing an assessment, that they have completed response plans, and each system must keep a copy of its plan for 5 years. Directs EPA to provide guidance to community water systems serving fewer than 3,300 individuals on how to conduct vulnerability assessments, prepare emergency response plans, and address threats. Authorizes $160 million for FY2002, and such sums as may be necessary for FY2003–FY2005, to provide financial assistance to community water systems to conduct assessments and prepare response plans, and to address basic security enhancements and significant threats. Security enhancements may include purchase and installation of intruder detection equipment and lighting, enhancing security of automated systems, personnel training and security screening. Authorizes EPA to use not more than $5 million of the funds to make grants to community water systems to assist in responding to and

Topic	Preexisting Law	P.L. 107-188
		alleviating any vulnerability to an attack or intentional act, which the Administrator determines to present an immediate and urgent security need. Further authorizes EPA to use not more than $5 million of the funds made available to make grants to community water systems serving fewer than 3,300 persons for activities and projects undertaken in accordance with the guidance for small systems that EPA must provide. [Section 401]
Contaminant prevention, detection, and response	No statutory provisions.	Adds a new Section 1434 to the SDWA directing the EPA Administrator, in consultation with CDC, and after consultation with other federal departments and state and local governments, to review (directly or through contracts or cooperative agreements) current and future methods to prevent, detect and respond to the intentional introduction of chemical, biological or radiological contaminants into community water systems and their source waters. The review must cover methods, means and equipment, including real time monitoring systems, for monitoring and detecting levels of contaminants; methods for providing sufficient notice to water system operators and those served by the system of the introduction of contaminants; methods, means and equipment for preventing the flow of contaminated water to people served by a system and for mitigating adverse effects on public health; methods and means for developing educational and awareness programs for water systems; and biomedical research on the public health impact of various contaminants that may be used in

Topic	Preexisting Law	P.L. 107-188
		attacks on water systems. Funding is authorized under Section 1435. [Section 402]
Supply disruption: prevention, detection and response	No statutory provisions.	Adds a new Section 1435 to the SDWA directing the EPA Administrator, in coordination with appropriate federal departments and agencies, to review methods and means by which terrorists or others could disrupt the drinking water supply or render it unsafe. This review must include a review of methods and means by which water systems could be destroyed, impaired, or made subject to cross-contamination, or by which information systems, including process controls, supervisory control and data acquisition (SCADA) and computer systems could be disrupted. EPA must also review methods and means by which systems could be reasonably protected from attacks, and by which alternative drinking water supplies could be provided if a water system was destroyed, impaired or contaminated. Requires EPA to ensure that these reviews reflect the needs of water systems of various sizes and geographic locations; EPA may consider the vulnerability of a specific region or service area, including the National Capital area. Directs EPA to share, as appropriate, the information developed under this section and Section 1434 with community water systems through the Information Sharing and Analysis Center (ISAC). Authorizes $15 million for FY2002, and such sums as may be necessary for FY2003–FY2005 to carry out Sections 1434 and 1435. [Section 402]

Topic	Preexisting Law	P.L. 107-188
Enforceable requirements	SDWA Section 1414(i)(1) identifies the sections of SDWA for which the Act's enforcement authorities apply.	Amends SDWA Section 1414(i)(1) to include a new Section 1433 requiring community water systems to conduct vulnerability assessments and to prepare emergency response plans, as an applicable and enforceable requirement under the Act. [Section 403]
Emergency powers	SDWA Section 1431 grants the EPA Administrator emergency powers to take such actions as deemed necessary to protect persons served by a public water system upon receipt of information that a contaminant that is present in, or is likely to enter, a public water system or an underground source of drinking water may present an imminent and substantial endangerment to health of those persons.	Amends SDWA Section 1431 to specify that EPA's emergency powers include the authority to act when there is a threatened or potential terrorist attack or other intentional act to disrupt the provision of safe drinking water or to impact the safety of a community's drinking water supply. [Section 403]
Penalties for tampering with public water systems	SDWA Section 1432 authorizes criminal and civil penalties for persons who tamper, attempt to tamper, or threaten to tamper with public water supplies. Provides that any person who tampers with a public water system shall be imprisoned for not more than 5 years, or fined, or both. Any person who attempts to tamper, or threatens to tamper, with a system shall be imprisoned for not more than 3 years. Provides that EPA may bring a civil action and that the appropriate federal court may impose a penalty of not more than $50,000 for tampering or not more than $20,000 for such attempt or threat.	Amends SDWA Section 1432 to increase criminal and civil penalties for tampering, attempting to tamper, or making threats to tamper with public water supplies. The maximum prison sentence for tampering is increased from 5 to 20 years. The maximum prison sentence for attempting to tamper, or making threats to tamper, is increased from 3 to 10 years. The maximum fine that may be imposed for tampering is increased from $50,000 to $1 million. The maximum fine for attempting to tamper, or threatening to tamper, is increased from $20,000 to $100,000. [Section 403]

Topic	Preexisting Law	P.L. 107-188
Technical assistance	SDWA Section 1442(b) authorizes EPA to provide technical assistance and to make grants to states and public water systems to assist in responding to and alleviating emergency situations.	Amends SDWA Section 1442(d) to authorize appropriations to carry out Section 1442(b) of not more than $35 million for FY2002, and such sums as may be necessary for each fiscal year thereafter. [Section 403]
Reauthorization of the Prescription Drug User Fee Act (FFDCA Sections 735–736)		
Types of fees	FFDCA Section 736(a) authorizes the Secretary to assess and collect three types of fees. First, a human drug application and supplement fee is due upon submission of the application or supplement. The Secretary may refund 75% of the fee if the application is not accepted. In the event the application is withdrawn after being filed, the Secretary may refund the fee or a portion of the fee if no substantial work was performed on it. The fee is waived for orphan drug applications and for supplements to drug applications that propose a new use for children. Second, annual establishment fees are assessed on each manufacturer of an approved drug for each fiscal year that an establishment manufactures the drug. Third, annual product fees are assessed on certain drugs registered under the FFDCA. Both establishment and product fees are due on Jan. 31 of each year.	Amends FFDCA Section 736(a) by requiring the annual establishment and product fees to be paid by October 1. Reduces by 50% the application and supplement fee for applications that contain no clinical data to review, and for filing a supplement. Eliminates the waiver for supplements for pediatric indications. Clarifies that the sponsor of the drug application is responsible for paying the annual product fee. Exempts from the product fee those products that are listed in the "Orange Book" with a potency described in terms of per 100mL, or which are the same as another approved products. [Section 504(a)]
Fee amounts	Under FFDCA Section 736(b), the application fee shall be $250,704 in FY1998, $256,338 in FY1999 and in FY2000, $267,606 in FY2001, and $258,451 in FY2002. The fee for an application that contains no clinical data to review, or for filing a supplement,	Amends FFDCA Section 736(b) by substituting a table setting out application/supplement, establishment, and product fee revenue, and total fee revenue, for FY2003 through FY2007. If subsequent legislation requires the Secretary to fund the additional costs of retirement of

Topic	Preexisting Law	P.L. 107-188
	is 50% of the application fee. Total establishment fee revenues shall be $35.6 million in FY1998, $36.4 million in FY1999 and in FY2000, $38 million in FY2001, and $36.7 million in FY2002. Total product fee revenues must equal the total establishment fee revenues.	federal personnel, fee revenue amounts may be increased to fully fund the portion of the added costs attributable to the process of review of drug applications. [Section 504(b)]
Fee adjustments	FFDCA Section 736(c) requires the Secretary each fiscal year to adjust fees and total fee revenues for inflation using either the average urban Consumer Price Index (CPI) or the increase in the civil service base pay for federal employees in Washington DC, whichever is greater. Each year's adjustment is added on a compounded basis to the sum of all the adjustments made for prior fiscal years. Requires the Secretary to adjust the annual establishment and product fees to ensure that the total amount collected equals that collected from application/supplement fees. Total fees collected for a fiscal year, as adjusted, may not exceed the total costs of reviewing drug applications for that year.	Amends FFDCA Section 736(c) as follows: (i) requires the inflation adjustment to use the CPI for the 12-month period ending June 30 of the year preceding the fiscal year for which the fees are being established or the civil service base pay as stated in the current law, whichever is greater; (ii) beginning in FY2004, creates a new workload adjustment (in addition to the inflation adjustment) to reflect changes in review workload; (iii) creates a new final year adjustment that permits the FDA, if necessary, to make a one-time fee increase in FY2007 to ensure that the agency has enough funds to operate for up to 3 months in FY2008 if there is a delay in reauthorizing PDUFA at the end of FY2007; and (iv) requires that the application/supplement, establishment, and product fees be established 60 days before the start of the fiscal year, based on the revenue amounts set out in Section 736(b) and the adjustments enumerated above. [Section 504(c)]
Fee waiver or reduction	FFDCA Section 736(d) permits the Secretary to reduce or waive one or more fees to protect public health or to remove barriers to innovation. Brand-name drug makers may seek a waiver if the fee would put them at an economic disadvantage relative	Amends FFDCA Section 736(d) by eliminating the waiver for brand-name drug manufacturers that claim the fee would put them at an economic disadvantage relative to generic drug producers. [Section 504(d)]

Topic	Preexisting Law	P.L. 107-188
	to a generic drug manufacturer. The Secretary may also waive the application fee for first-time drug applications from small businesses with fewer than 500 employees.	
Assessment of fees	Under FFDCA Section 736(f), fees may only be assessed for a fiscal year if the FDA's annual appropriation for salaries and expenses for that year is equal to or greater than its FY1997 appropriation, multiplied by whichever inflation adjustment factor is applicable for the fiscal year in question. This "trigger" ensures that PDUFA fees are not a substitute for the agency's annual appropriations.	Changes the title of Section 736(f) but leaves the trigger as is. [Section 504(e)]
Crediting and availability of fees	FFDCA Section 736(g) permits FDA to transfer collected fees to its salaries and expenses account, without fiscal year limitation, to be used solely for reviewing drug applications. Fees must be collected in an amount equal to that specified in the annual appropriations act and may only be collected and available to defray the increase in application review costs over the costs for such activities in FY1997, adjusted for inflation. This second "trigger" is intended to ensure that PDUFA fees are used to accelerate the drug application review process and not substitute for "normal level" expenses. Authorizes the following appropriations for fees: $106.8 million for FY1997; $109.2 million for FY1999 and for FY2000; $114 million for FY2001; and $110.1 million for FY2002, adjusting as	Amends FFDCA Section 736(g) by providing FDA a 5% margin of error for meeting the requirements of the second trigger. The intent of this modification is to relieve FDA of the need to overspend each year, which the agency has done consistently to ensure that its expenditures do not fall below the trigger amount and cause it to lose the authority to collect fees. Authorizes the following appropriations for fees: $222.9 million for FY2003; $231million for FY2004; $252 million for FY2005; $259.3 million for FY2006; and $259.3 million for FY2007, adjusting as specified above. [Section 504(f)]

Topic	Preexisting Law	P.L. 107-188
	specified above. Collected fees that exceed the authorized amount must be subtracted from the amount of fees authorized to be collected in the subsequent fiscal year.	
Accountability and reports	The Food and Drug Administration Modernization Act of 1997 (FDAMA; P.L. 105-115, Section 104) required the Secretary to provide Congress with an annual performance report and an annual fiscal report.	Requires the Secretary to consult with Congress and interested public and private stakeholders in developing recommendations for the next PDUFA reauthorization. Requires the Secretary to publish the recommendations in the *Federal Register* for public comment. Requires the Secretary to provide Congress with an annual performance report and an annual fiscal report [Section 505]
Reports of postmarketing studies	FFDCA Section 506B establishes annual reporting requirements for drug sponsors who enter into agreements with the Secretary to conduct a postmarketing study.	Amends FFDCA Section 506B to require the Secretary, in the event a sponsor fails to complete an agreed upon study, to post a statement on the FDA's Web site to that effect. Give the Secretary the authority to require sponsors who fail to complete studies of fast-track drugs and biological products for serious and life-threatening illnesses to notify health care practitioners of the sponsor's failure to complete the study and of unanswered questions relating to the clinical benefits and safety of the product. [Section 506]
Effective date and sunset	FDAMA Sections 106–107 reauthorized PDUFA from October 1, 1997 through September 30, 2002, with required annual reports due no later than 120 days thereafter.	The amendments made by this subtitle take effect on October 1, 2002, and sunset on September 30, 2007. The annual reporting requirements of Section 505 remain effective for an additional 120 days. [Sections 508–509]

Topic	Preexisting Law	P.L. 107-188
Miscellaneous Provisions		
Digital television	Section 201 of the Telecommunications Act of 1996 (P.L. 104-104) provided that digital television licenses issued by the Federal Communications Commission (FCC) should be limited to existing broadcasters. On April 3, 1997, the FCC allotted digital television spectrum to all eligible broadcasters existing at that time.	Requires the FCC to allot a digital channel to any requesting full-power television station that had an application pending for an analog television station construction permit as of October 24, 1991, and which had its application granted after April 3, 1997. Any station receiving digital spectrum under this provision is required to complete construction of its digital facility within 18 months, without the possibility of an extension. Stations are also prohibited from operating an analog signal on their designated digital channel. [Section 531]
Medicare + Choice	Section 1853 of the Social Security Act (SSA) requires the Centers for Medicare and Medicaid Services (CMS) to announce the annual Medicare + Choice (M+C) payment rates on March 1 of each year that will be applicable on January 1 of the following year. Section 1854 requires that each M+C organization must submit to the Secretary for approval, for each of its M+C plans, specific information about the adjusted community rate (ACR), M+C premiums, cost sharing, and additional benefits (if any) no later than July 1 of each year, also for the following year. Section 1851 permits individuals to make and change election to an M+C plan on an ongoing basis. Beginning in 2002, elections and changes to elections are available on a more limited basis. Individuals can make or change elections each November, during the	Moves the CMS annual announcement of M+C payment rates from no later than March 1 to no later than the second Monday in May, effective only in 2003 and 2004. Moves the deadline for plans to submit information about ACRs, M+C premiums, cost sharing, and additional benefits (if any) from no later than July 1 to no later than the second Monday in September in 2002, 2003, and 2004. Changes the annual coordinated election period from the month of November to November 15 – December 31 in 2002, 2003, and 2004. Allows Medicare beneficiaries to make and change election to an M+C plan on an ongoing basis through 2004. Beginning in 2005, individuals would only be able to make changes on the more limited basis, originally scheduled to be phased in beginning in 2002. [Section 532]

Topic	Preexisting Law	P.L. 107-188
	annual coordinated election period. Current Medicare beneficiaries may also change their election at any time during the first 6 months of 2002 (or first 3 months of any subsequent year). Special enrollment rules apply to newly eligible aged beneficiaries. Special enrollment periods apply to enrollees under limited situations, such as a change in place of residence.	

APPENDIX A. BIOTERRORISM-RELATED HEARINGS 107TH CONGRESS

Senate Appropriations Subcommittee on Labor, HHS, and Education

October 3, 2001	Bioterrorism: Public health preparedness and response
October 23, 2001	Public health response to anthrax attack
November 2, 2001	Smallpox: Public health preparedness and response
November 29, 2001	Funding for bioterrorism preparedness

Senate Appropriations Subcommittee on VA-HUD and Independent Agencies

November 28, 2001	Anthrax decontamination

Senate Armed Services Subcommittee on Emerging Threats and Capabilities

October 25, 2001	Bioterrorism and the Dark Winter exercise

Senate Commerce, Science and Transportation Committee

February 5, 2002	Bioterrorism: Countermeasures R&D (Subcommittee on Science, Technology, and Space)

Senate Environment and Public Works Committee

December 4, 2001	Anthrax decontamination

Senate Foreign Relations Committee

September 5, 2001	Bioterrorism threat and the spread of infectious diseases

Senate Governmental Affairs Committee

July 23, 2001	Bioterrorism: FEMA's role and public health preparedness (Subcommittee on National Security, Proliferation and Federal Services)
October 17, 2001	Bioterrorism: Federal agency preparedness
October 30-31, 2001	Anthrax in the mail: Protecting postal workers and the public
April 18, 2002	Public health preparedness

Senate Health, Education, Labor, and Pensions Committee

September 26, 2001	Psychological trauma of terrorism
October 9, 2001	Bioterrorism: Public health preparedness and response
November 2, 2001	Kids and terrorism (Subcommittee on Children and Families)

Senate Judiciary Committee

November 6, 2001	Law enforcement and the domestic bioterrorism threat (Subcommittee on Technology, Terrorism and Government Information)

House Appropriations Subcommittee on Labor, HHS, and Education

May 1, 2002	HHS bioterrorism preparedness

House Energy and Commerce Committee

October 10, 2001	Bioterrorism preparedness and response (Subcommittee on Oversight and Investigations)
November 1, 2001	Public health early-warning surveillance systems (Subcommittee on Oversight and Investigations)
November 7, 2001	Physical security and NIH and CDC facilities (Subcommittee on Oversight and Investigations)
November 15, 2001	Bioterrorism: Public health preparedness and response

House Government Reform Committee

May 1, 2001	Management of medical stockpiles (Subcommittee on National Security, Veterans Affairs and International Relations)
July 23, 2001	Federal response to a bioterrorism attack: Dark Winter (Subcommittee on National Security, Veterans Affairs and International Relations)
October 5, 2001	Bioterrorism: Federal, state, and local preparedness (Subcommittee on Government Efficiency, Financial Management and Intergovernmental Relations)
October 12, 2001	Assessing the threat of bioterrorism (Subcommittee on National Security, Veterans Affairs and International Relations)
October 23, 2001	Vaccine research and development (Subcommittee on National Security, Veterans Affairs and International Relations)
October 30, 2001	Anthrax and postal worker safety

November 7, 2001	DOD medical readiness for chemical and biological warfare (Subcommittee on National Security, Veterans Affairs and International Relations)
November 14, 2001	Medical care for bioterrorism victims
November 29, 2001	Risk communication: National security and public health (Subcommittee on National Security, Veterans Affairs and International Relations)
December 14, 2001	Bioterrorism response: Information sharing between local, state, and federal governments (Subcommittee on Technology and Procurement Policy)
February 28, 2002	Anthrax antitoxin research
March 1, 2002	Federal, state, and local response to biological and chemical attack (Subcommittee on Government Efficiency, Financial Management and Intergovernmental Relations)
March 21, 2002	Combating terrorism (Subcommittee on National Security, Veterans Affairs and International Relations)

House International Relations Committee

December 5, 2001	Bioterrorism and potential sources of anthrax

House Science Committee

November 8, 2001	Anthrax decontamination
December 5, 2001	Bioterrorism: Federal preparedness and response

House Veterans' Affairs Committee

April 10, 2002	Bioterrorism legislation (H.R. 3253, H.R. 3254)

Appendix B. Bioterrorism-Related Web Sites

Department of Health and Human Services

Information on public health preparedness	[http://www.hhs.gov/hottopics/healing]
DHHS Office of Emergency Preparedness	[http://www.oep.dhhs.gov]
DHHS Office of Public Health Preparedness	[http://www.hhs.gov/ophp]
Metropolitan Medical Response Systems	[http://www.mmrs.hhs.gov]
National Pharmaceutical Stockpile Program	[http://www.cdc.gov/nceh/nps/default.htm]
Centers for Disease Control and Prevention	[http://www.bt.cdc.gov]
Health Resources and Services Admin.	[http://www.hrsa.gov/bioterrorism.htm]
Food and Drug Administration	[http://www.fda.gov/oc/opacom/hottopics/bioterrorism.html]
National Institutes of Health	[http://www.niaid.nih.gov/publications/bioterrorism.htm]
National Library of Medicine	[http://www.nlm.nih.gov/medlineplus/biologicalandchemicalweapons.html]

Department of Defense

U.S. Army Medical Research Institute of Infectious Diseases	[http://www.usamriid.army.mil]
DOD Anthrax Vaccine Immunization Program	[http://www.anthrax.osd.mil]
Nuclear, Biological, Chemical Medical Reference Site	[http://www.nbc-med.org/others]

State and Local Health Departments

Many health departments have included information on bioterrorism and public health preparedness on their Web sites. For links to state and local health departments, go to [http://www.apha.org/state_local/afflinks.htm].

Professional Associations

American College of Emergency Physicians	[http://www.acep.org/1,4634,0.html]
American College of Physicians	[http://www.acponline.org/bioterro]
American Hospital Association	[http://www.hospitalconnect.com/aha/key_issues/disaster_readiness/index.html]
American Medical Association	[http://www.ama-assn.org/ama/pub/category/6671.html]
American Society for Microbiology	[http://www.asmusa.org/pasrc/bioprep.htm]
Association for Professionals in Infection Control and Epidemiology	[http://www.apic.org/bioterror]
Association of State and Territorial Health Officials	[http://www.astho.org]
Council of State and Territorial Epidemiologists	[http://www.cste.org]
Federation of American Scientists, Chemical & Biological Arms Control Program	[http://fas.org/bwc/index.html]
Nat. Assoc. of County & City Health Officials	[http://www.naccho.org/files/documents/responds_to_bioterrorism.html]

Academic Resources

Johns Hopkins Center for Civilian Biodefense Studies	[http://www.hopkins-biodefense.org]
The Henry L. Stimson Center	[http://www.stimson.org/cbw]
Monterey Institute of International Studies	[http://www.cns.miis.edu]
Chemical and Biological Arms Control Institute	[http://www.cbaci.org]
UCLA Center for Public Health and Disaster Relief	[http://www.ph.ucla.edu/cphdr]
University of Minnesota Center for Infectious Disease Research and Policy	[http://www1.umn.edu/cidrap]
St. Louis University Center for the Study of Bioterrorism and Emerging Infections	[http://bioterrorism.slu.edu]
Columbia University Center for Public Health Preparedness	[http://cpmcnet.columbia.edu/dept/sph/CPHP/index.html]
University of North Carolina Center for Public Health Preparedness	[http://www.sph.unc.edu/bioterrorism]

Chapter 2

BIOTERRORISM: LEGISLATION TO IMPROVE PUBLIC HEALTH PREPAREDNESS AND RESPONSE CAPACITY[•]

C. Stephen Redhead, Donna U. Vogt and Mary E. Tiemann

SUMMARY

The recent anthrax attacks, though small in scale compared to the scenarios envisioned by bioterrorism experts, strained the public health system and raised concern that the nation is insufficiently prepared to respond to bioterrorist attacks. Improving public health preparedness and response capacity offers protection not only from bioterrorist attacks, but also from naturally occurring public health emergencies.

In December 2001, the House and Senate each passed legislation (H.R. 3448, S. 1765) to improve the public health system's capacity to respond to bioterrorism. This legislation builds on the programs and authorities established in Title III of the Public Health Service (PHS) Act by the Public Health Threats and Emergencies Act of 2000 (P.L. 106-505, Title I). While the two bills are similar in many respects, there are several key differences that are being addressed in conference.

The Senate bill (S. 1765) would authorize a total of \$3.25 billion in FY2002 to increase the public health system's bioterrorism preparedness and response capability, including \$640 million to expand the National Pharmaceutical Stockpile (NPS), \$509 million to purchase smallpox vaccine, and \$1.46 billion for grants to state and local health departments and hospitals. S. 1765 would also strengthen regulation of domestic and imported food by the Food and Drug Administration (FDA) and give the U.S. Department of Agriculture (USDA) new authority to safeguard the nation's agricultural industry from the threat of bioterrorism.

The House bill (H.R. 3448) would authorize almost \$3 billion in FY2002 for bioterrorism preparedness, including \$646 million to expand the NPS, \$509 million to purchase smallpox vaccine, and \$1 billion for grants to states and localities. H.R. 3448 does not include any of the agricultural provisions that appear in S. 1765. Unlike the Senate bill, however, H.R. 3448

[•] Excerpted from CRS Report

includes provisions to protect community drinking water supplies from bioterrorism and it places more emphasis on upgrading facilities at the Centers for Disease Control and Prevention (CDC).

While lawmakers work towards final passage of new authorizing legislation, Congress has appropriated $3 billion to the Dept. of Health and Human Services (HHS) for FY2002 to increase bioterrorism preparedness at the federal, state, and local levels. HHS anti-bioterrorism funding was included in the FY2002 Labor-HHS-Education appropriations bill (P.L. 107-116, H.R. 3061) and in the $20 billion emergency spending package (P.L. 107-117, H.R. 3338). HHS is dispersing the funds according to existing authorities and the broad spending parameters set out in the appropriations bills.

INTRODUCTION

The September 11, 2001 terrorist attacks and the subsequent deliberate release of anthrax spores in the mail have focused policymakers' attention on the preparedness and response capability of the U.S. public health system. Though small in scale compared to the scenarios envisioned by bioterrorism experts and played out in recent government exercises, the recent anthrax attacks strained the public health system and exposed weaknesses at the federal, state, and local levels. Many bioterrorism experts believe that had those responsible for the anthrax attacks employed a more sophisticated delivery mechanism or released a deadly communicable biological agent such as smallpox, the health care system may have been overwhelmed.

Bioterrorism poses a unique challenge to the medical care and public health systems. Unlike an explosion or chemical attack, which results in immediate and visible casualties, the public health impact of a biological attack can unfold gradually over time. Until a sufficient number of people arrive at emergency rooms and doctors' offices complaining of similar illnesses, there may be no sign that an attack has taken place. The speed and accuracy with which doctors and laboratories reach the correct diagnoses and report their findings to public health authorities has a direct impact on the number of people who become ill and the number that die. The nation's ability to respond to a bioterrorist attack, therefore, depends crucially on the state of preparedness of its medical care systems and public health infrastructure.

Public health experts have for years complained about the deterioration of the public health system through neglect and lack of funding. They warn that the nation is ill-equipped and insufficiently prepared to respond to a bioterrorist attack. For example, they point out that there are too few medical personnel trained to spot biological attacks, a shortage of sophisticated laboratories to identify the agents, and inadequate supplies of drugs and vaccines to counteract the threat. They also contend that inadequate plans exist for setting up quarantines and emergency facilities to handle the sick and infectious victims. Improving public health preparedness and response capacity offers protection not only from bioterrorist attacks, but also from naturally occurring public health emergencies. Public health officials are increasingly concerned about our exposure and susceptibility to infectious disease and food-borne illness because of global travel, ubiquitous food imports, and the evolution of antibiotic-resistant pathogens.

In December 2001, the House and Senate each passed comprehensive bioterrorism preparedness legislation (H.R. 3448, S. 1765) with broad bipartisan support. This chapter summarizes H.R. 3448 and S. 1765 and provides a side-by-side comparison of the provisions in each bill and in current law. Lawmakers also appropriated $3 billion to the Dept. of Health and Human Services (HHS) for FY2002 to improve bioterrorism preparedness. Anti-bioterrorism funding was provided in the FY2002 Labor-HHS-Education appropriations bill (P.L. 107-116, H.R. 3061) and in the anti-terrorism emergency supplemental appropriations bill (P.L. 107-117, H.R. 3338). Details of HHS's bioterrorism funding, including the Administration's FY2003 budget request, are provided in Appendix A. Appendix B provides information on the HHS grant programs to improve public health and hospital preparedness. Appendix C lists all the bioterrorism-related hearings in the 107th Congress. In most cases, hearing testimony is available on the committee Web sites. Finally, Appendix D provides a list of bioterrorism-related Web sites.

HOUSE AND SENATE BIOTERRORISM LEGISLATION

Bioterrorism Preparedness Act (S. 1765)

Senators Frist and Kennedy introduced the Bioterrorism Preparedness Act (S. 1715) on November 15, 2001. In a procedural move aimed at bypassing committee consideration and allowing prompt floor consideration, the legislation's sponsors reintroduced the bill (S. 1765) with 74 cosponsors on December 4, 2001. On December 20,2001, the Senate took up the House bioterrorism bill (H.R. 3448, see below), substituted the text of S. 1765, and passed H.R. 3448, as amended.

The Bioterrorism Preparedness Act builds on the programs and authorities established in Title III of the Public Health Service (PHS) Act by the Public Health Threats and Emergencies Act of 2000 (P.L. 106-505, Title I). S. 1765 incorporates ideas and objectives from a number of other Senate bioterrorism bills introduced in the wake of the anthrax attacks.[1] It is intended to improve the health system's capacity to respond to bioterrorism, protect the nation's food supply from bioterrorist attacks, speed the development and production of new drug treatments and vaccines, improve coordination of federal anti-bioterrorism activities, and increase investment in state and local preparedness. S. 1765 is a 5-year authorization bill, which calls for a total of $3.25 billion in funding for FY2002 and such sums as may be necessary for the remaining years. Key provisions of the bill are summarized in the text box below, including the authorized appropriations for FY2002 (in parentheses).

[1] Senate bioterrorism preparedness bills introduced in response to the September 11 attacks and the anthrax incidents include: the Biological and Chemical Weapons Preparedness Act of 2001 (S. 1486) introduced by Senator Edwards on Oct. 3, 2001; the Biological and Chemical Attack Preparedness Act (S. 1508) introduced by Senator Corzine on Oct. 4, 2001; the State Bioterrorism Preparedness Act (S. 1520) introduced by Senator Bayh on Oct. 9, 2001; the Protecting America's Children Against Terrorism Act (S. 1539) introduced by Senator Clinton on Oct. 11,2001; the Bioterrorism Awareness Act (S. 1548) introduced by Senator Carnahan on Oct. 15,2001; the Protecting the Food Supply from Bioterrorism Act (S. 1551) introduced by Senator Clinton on Oct. 15, 2001; the Agricultural Bioterrorism Countermeasures Act of 2001 (S. 1563) introduced by Senator Hutchison on Oct. 17,2001; the Public Health Emergency Planning and Information Act of 2001 (S. 1574) introduced by Senator Rockefeller on Oct. 25,2001; the Pathogen Research, Emergency Preparedness and Response Efforts (PREPARE) Act of 2001 (S. 1635) introduced by Senator Hutchinson on Nov. 6,2001; and the Deadly Biological Agent Control Act of 2001 (S. 1661) introduced by Senator Feinstein on Nov. 8, 2001.

Bioterrorism Preparedness Act of 2001 (S. 1765)

I. Federal Bioterrorism Preparedness and Response Capability:
- Expand the National Pharmaceutical Stockpile ($640 million).
- Upgrade CDC's bioterrorism response capability ($60 million).
- Improve public health laboratories ($59.5 million).
- Tighten controls on the possession and use of biological agents and toxins.

II. State and Local Bioterrorism Preparedness and Response Capability:
- Authorize block grants to states ($667 million).
- Expand existing discretionary grant programs ($420 million).
- Authorize grants to improve hospital response capability ($370 million).

III. Anti-Bioterrorism Drugs and Vaccines:
- Purchase smallpox vaccine ($509 million).
- Authorize long-term contracts for vaccine and drug development and provide limited exemption from federal antitrust laws.

IV. Food Supply and Agriculture ($525.5 million):
- Strengthen FDA regulation of domestic and imported food.
- Expand and upgrade the safety and security of the nation's food supply, livestock, and crops.

Public Health Security and Bioterrorism Response Act (H.R. 3448)

Representatives Tauzin (R-LA) and Dingell (D-MI) introduced the Public Health Security and Bioterrorism Response Act (H.R. 3448) on December 11,2001. The bill was immediately considered under suspension of the rules and passed by the House the following day on a vote of 418–2 In many respects, H.R. 3448, which authorizes $3 billion in FY2002 to improve bioterrorism preparedness and response capacity, resembles the Senate-passed bill. Both bills would authorize funds to expand the National Pharmaceutical Stockpile, purchase smallpox vaccine, develop and produce anthrax vaccine, and provide grants to state and local governments and public health departments. However, there are a number of key differences between the House and Senate bills that are being addressed in conference.

S. 1765 contains several provisions aimed at combating agricultural terrorism, including one that would authorize the creation of a surveillance and response system to detect biological threats to animals and plants. Another provision would authorize the Secretary of Agriculture to award grants to universities to conduct research on improving the security of facilities at which hazardous biological agents and toxins are stored for agricultural research purposes. H.R. 3448 does not include any agricultural provisions. The Senate bill also provides a limited exemption from federal antitrust law that would enable drug companies to collaborate to develop vaccines. The House version has no such provision.

H.R. 3448 includes a set of provisions aimed at protecting the nation's drinking water supply, which are not included in S. 1765. The House bill would authorize a total of $170 million in FY2002 to assess the vulnerability of community drinking water systems, help communities develop emergency response plans, and take other steps to protect the water supply from acts of terrorism. H.R. 3448 also contains language that would strengthen FDA regulation of imported drugs, which is not present in S. 1765, and it places more emphasis on upgrading CDC's facilities and capacities. Key provisions of the House bill are summarized in the text box below, including the authorized appropriations for FY2002 (in parentheses).

Public Health Security and Bioterrorism Response Act of 2001 (H.R. 3448)

I. Federal Bioterrorism Preparedness and Response Capacity:
- Expand the National Pharmaceutical Stockpile ($646 million).
- Upgrade CDC's bioterrorism response capacity ($450 million).
- Tighten controls on the possession and use of biological agents and toxins.

II. State and Local Bioterrorism Preparedness and Response Capacity:
- Expand existing discretionary grant programs ($910 million).
- Relieve shortages of critical health care professionals ($40 million).

III. Anti-Bioterrorism Drugs and Vaccines:
- Purchase smallpox vaccine ($509 million).
- Stockpile potassium iodide near nuclear power plants.

IV. Food and Drug Supply:
- Strengthen FDA regulation of domestic and imported food ($100 million).
- Strengthen FDA regulation of imported drugs.

V. Drinking Water:
- Upgrade safety and security of drinking water supplies ($170 million).

Table 1 provides a side-by-side comparison of H.R. 3448, S. 1765, and, where applicable, current law. All the PHS Act Title III provisions relating to public health emergencies that were established by P.L. 106-505 (i.e., Sections 319, 319A–319G) are included in the table, regardless of whether they are amended by S. 1765 or H.R. 3448.

Table 1. Side-by-Side Comparison of Legislation on Public Health Preparedness for Bioterrorism

Topic	Current Law	S. 1765 Frist/Kennedy	H.R. 3448 Tauzin/Dingell
Establishing National Goals and Public Health Capacities, Assessing Public Health Needs			
Establishing National Goals, Reports to Congress	No statutory provisions.	Adds a new Title XXVIII to the Public Health Service (PHS) Act setting out the following national goals for bioterrorism preparedness: (i) provide federal assistance to states and localities in the event of an attack; (ii) improve public health preparedness and response; (iii) develop new vaccines and therapies; (iv) protect the food supply and agriculture. [Section 101] Adds a new Section 2811 to the PHS Act to require the Secretary to report to Congress within 1 year, and biennially thereafter, on progress made toward meeting the objectives of the Act, including recommendations for new legislative authority needed to protect public health. Requires the Secretary to report to Congress within 1 year on the vulnerability of rural communities to bioterrorism and recommend any new legislative authority needed to strengthen the preparedness of such communities. [Section 201]	Adds a new Title XXVIII to the Public Health Service (PHS) Act that requires the Secretary, building on existing authority in PHS Act Section 319A, to develop and implement a bioterrorism preparedness and response plan, in consultation with other federal agencies. The plan would coordinate the activities of state and local governments and meet the preparedness goals in the bill (e.g., effective assistance to state and local governments, laboratory readiness, effective communications networks, training, and surveillance). Requires the Secretary to evaluate the feasibility of utilizing the Dept. of Veterans Affairs' research capabilities. Similar reporting requirements to those in S. 1765. [Section 101]
Establishing Public Health Capacities	Public Health Service (PHS) Act Section 319A requires the Secretary, together with state and local health	No provisions.	No provisions.

Topic	Current Law	S. 1765 Frist/Kennedy	H.R. 3448 Tauzin/Dingell
	officials, to establish what capacities are needed for national, state, and local public health systems to be able to detect, diagnose, and contain outbreaks of infectious disease, drug-resistant pathogens, or acts of bioterrorism. Authorizes $4 million for FY2001 and such sums as may be necessary for FY2002–FY2006.		
Assessing Public Health Needs	PHS Act Section 319B authorizes grants to states and local public health departments to evaluate the extent to which they can achieve the capacities identified pursuant to Section 319A. Requires the Secretary to develop a national framework for the evaluations. Authorizes $45 million for FY2001, and such sums as may be necessary for FY2002–FY2003.	No provisions.	No provisions.
Federal (HHS) Preparedness and Response Capacity			
Assistant Secretary for Emergency Preparedness	No statutory provisions.	Adds a new Section 2813 to the PHS Act authorizing the appointment of an Assistant Secretary for Emergency Preparedness to head the Office of Emergency Preparedness and coordinate all HHS bioterrorism activities. [Section 211]	Adds a new Section 2811 to the PHS Act authorizing the appointment of an Assistant Secretary for Emergency Preparedness to coordinate all HHS bioterrorism-related activities under the Act and interface with other federal agencies. [Section 102]
Public Health Emergencies	PHS Act Section 319 authorizes the Secretary to respond to public health	Amends PHS Act Section 319 to require the Secretary to notify Congress within	Amends PHS Act Section 319 as follows: (i) permits the Secretary

Topic	Current Law	S. 1765 Frist/Kennedy	H.R. 3448 Tauzin/Dingell
	emergencies, including diseases, disorders, or bioterrorist attacks, by supporting grants, contracts, and investigations. Establishes the Public Health Emergency Fund and authorizes such sums as may be necessary. Requires an annual report to Congress on expenditures from the Fund.	48 hours of declaring a public health emergency. Allows such a declaration to remain in effect for 180 days and permits the Secretary to extend that period, provided Congress is notified within 48 hours of the extension. Allows the Secretary, as a result of public health emergencies, to waive deadlines for the submission of data and reports by individuals or public or private entities pursuant to any law administered by the Secretary. [Section 212]	during a public health emergency to transfer funds between appropriations accounts administered under this Act, without lengthy waiting periods, and requires the Secretary to notify Congress of the intent to make such a transfer; and (ii) provides that public health emergencies expire by announcement of the Secretary or after 90 days, whichever comes first, and permits the Secretary to renew emergency declarations. Similar waiver authority to S. 1765. [Section 131, 134]
Quarantine and Inspection	PHS Act Section 361 authorizes the Surgeon General, in consultation with the Secretary, to develop quarantine, inspection, fumigation, sanitation, and pest extermination regulations to prevent the introduction, transmission, or spread of communicable diseases. Section 363 authorizes the development of regulations for the apprehension and examination of infected individuals in times of war.	No provisions.	Amends PHS Act Secs. 361 and 363 by eliminating the prerequisite for a National Advisory Health Council recommendation before issuing a quarantine rule or a rule providing for the apprehension of individuals during wartime. Permits federal regulations under Secs. 361 & 363, as amended, to preempt state laws that conflict with the exercise of federal authority. [Section 132]
Federal Working Groups and Advisory Committees	PHS Act Section 319F requires the Secretary to: (i) establish, with the Secretary of Defense, an interagency working group on bioterrorism preparedness, and (ii) establish, in	Amends PHS Act Section 319F by eliminating the two existing working groups and replacing them with a single interagency working group on the prevention, preparedness, and response	Amends PHS Act Section 319Fby expanding the composition and responsibilities of the two existing interagency working groups. Requires the Secretary to establish the

Topic	Current Law	S. 1765 Frist/Kennedy	H.R. 3448 Tauzin/Dingell
	collaboration with the Director of FEMA, the Attorney General, and the Secretary of Agriculture, an interagency working group to address the public health and medical consequences of a bioterrorist attack.	to bioterrorism, to be established by the Secretary in coordination with the Director of FEMA, the Attorney General, and the Secretaries of Agriculture, Defense, Labor, and Veterans Affairs (VA), and with other federal officials as appropriate. Creates two advisory committees to the Secretary: (i) the National Task Force on Children and Terrorism; and (ii) the Emergency Public Information and Communications Task Force. Both Task Forces sunset after 1 year. [Section 213]	preparedness working group in coordination with the Director of FEMA, the Attorney General, the Secretaries of Agriculture, Defense, Energy, and the VA, and the EPA Administrator. Requires the Secretary to establish the public health and medical working group in coordination with the Director of FEMA, the Attorney General, the Secretaries of Agriculture, Defense, Labor, and the VA, and the EPA Administrator. Creates two advisory committees to the Secretary: (i) the National Advisory Committee on Children and Terrorism; and (ii) the Emergency Public Information and Communications Advisory Committee. Both committees sunset after 1 year. Requires a coordinated strategy on public health communications during a bioterrorist attack. [Section 104,108]
National Disaster Medical System (NDMS)	No statutory provisions. The NDMS was established in 1984 as a partnership of four federal agencies (HHS, FEMA, DOD, VA), state and local governments, and the private sector to provide medical assistance and hospitalization for mass casualties	Adds a new Section 2814 to the PHS Act providing statutory authorization for the NDMS, to be coordinated by the Secretary in collaboration with FEMA, DOD, and the VA. Appoints activated NDMS volunteers as temporary federal employees and establishes employment	Adds a new Section 2811 to the PHS Act containing similar provisions to S. 1765, but with the following additional requirements and authorizations: requires the Secretary to collaborate with states and other public and private entities, and, within

Topic	Current Law	S. 1765 Frist/Kennedy	H.R. 3448 Tauzin/Dingell
	in the event of a natural or man-made disaster. It consists of more than 7,000 volunteer health professionals and support personnel. For more information, go to [http://ndms.dhhs.gov].	and reemployment rights for NDMS volunteers. [Section 211]	1 year and periodically thereafter, to conduct exercises to test the capability and timeliness of the NDMS. Requires the Secretary to establish education and training criteria for NDMS personnel. Authorizes such sums as may be necessary for FY2002–FY2006 for NDMS and to provide for the Assistant Secretary of Emergency Preparedness. [Section 102]
National Pharmaceutical Stockpile (NPS)	No statutory provisions. The NPS, which was established and is managed by the CDC, includes pharmaceuticals, vaccines, and medical supplies that can be deployed anywhere in the country in response to a public health emergency. For more information, go to [http://www.cdc.gov/nceh/nps/default.htm].	Adds a new Section 2812 to the PHS Act requiring the Secretary, in coordination with the VA Secretary, to maintain a National Pharmaceutical Stockpile of vaccines, drugs, medical devices and supplies to meet the nation's emergency public health needs. Authorizes $640 million for FY2002, and such sums as may be necessary for FY2003–2006. [Section 201]	Similar provisions to S. 1765, but with additional requirements for periodic review of the stockpile and the development of a distribution plan. Requires the Secretary to consult with the Director of FEMA, the Attorney General, the Secretaries of Agriculture, DOD, Energy, and the VA, the EPA Administrator, and state and local agencies. Authorizes $1.155 billion for FY2002, of which $509 million is for purchasing smallpox vaccine, and such sums as may be necessary for FY2003–2006. [Section 121, 151]
Upgrading CDC	PHS Act Section 319D authorizes funds for the construction and renovation of CDC facilities, and to support the agency's activities to combat threats to public health.	Amends PHS Act Section 319D to clarify CDC's role in responding to bioterrorism. Authorizes $60 million for FY2002, and such sum as may be necessary for FY2003–FY2006, to	Amends PHS Act Section 319D to clarify CDC's role in responding to bioterrorism. Requires the Secretary to upgrade CDC's facilities and capacities. Provides authorization and

Topic	Current Law	S. 1765 Frist/Kennedy	H.R. 3448 Tauzin/Dingell
	Authorizes $180 million for FY2001, and such sums as may be necessary for FY2002–FY2010.	upgrade CDC's facilities and capacities. [Section 202]	multi-year contracting authority for renovation, development, and security at CDC facilities. Authorizes $450 million for FY2002, of which $300 million is for upgrading facilities, $300 million for FY2003 to upgrade facilities, and such sums as may be necessary for FY2004–FY2006. [Section 103,151]
Public Health Laboratories Network, National Public Health Communications and Surveillance Network	No statutory provisions. Over the past 3 years, CDC has awarded grants to all 50 states and some metropolitan health departments to enhance state and local laboratory capacity and to help build an national electronic communications network connecting all the components of the public health community. For more information, go to [http://www.bt.cdc.gov].	Amends PHS Act Section 319D to provide grants to establish a coordinated network of public health labs. Authorizes $59.5 million for FY2002, and such sums as may be necessary for FY2003–FY2006. [Section 202]	Amends PHS Act Section 319D to provide grants to establish a coordinated network of public health labs and to develop a national public health communications and surveillance network. Authorizes such sums as necessary for FY2002–FY2006. [Section 103] Requires that all the FY2003 and FY2004 infrastructure grants provided by the National Telecommunications and Information Administration be awarded to health providers to facilitate participation in the national public health communications and surveillance network. [Section 139]
Education and Training of Health Care Personnel: Children and Other Vulnerable	PHS Act 319F requires the Secretary to develop programs to educate health professionals in recognizing and caring for victims of bioterrorist attacks and programs to train laboratory personnel	Amends PHS Act Section 319F to require the interagency working group on the public health and medical consequences of bioterrorism, in collaboration with professional	Amends PHS Act Section 319F by requiring the Secretary, in collaboration with the interagency working group and professional organizations, to award grants for the

Topic	Current Law	S. 1765 Frist/Kennedy	H.R. 3448 Tauzin/Dingell
Populations	in identifying bioweapons.	organizations, to develop education programs that recognize the special needs of children and other vulnerable populations during public health emergencies. [Section 313; Note: The interagency working group to which this subsection of the Act refers would be replaced by two advisory committees under S. 1765, see above.]	development of education materials to teach health officials and other emergency personnel to identify potential bioweapons and care for victims, recognizing the special needs of children and other vulnerable populations during public health emergencies. [Section 105]
GAO Report	PHS Act 319F requires a GAO report to Congress, within 6 months, on federal bioterrorism-related activities, including research, preparedness, and response. [This report, GAO-01-915, was issued by GAO on September 28, 2001.]	Amends PHS Act Section 319F to require a new GAO report to Congress on federal bioterrorism-related activities, including the development of public health lab capacity. [Section 314]	No provisions.
Occupational Safety and Health	Section 22 of the Occupational Safety and Health Act of 1970 (29 U.S.C. 671) created the National Institute for Occupational Safety and Health (NIOSH) as the federal agency responsible for conducting research and making recommendations for the prevention of work-related disease and injury. NIOSH is part of the CDC.	Amends OSH Act Section 22 to expand NIOSH research on bioterrorism threats and attacks in the workplace. [Section 315]	Requires the Secretary, acting through the Director of NIOSH, to expand research on bioterrorism threats and attacks in the workplace. [Section 138]
Agency for Toxic Substances and Disease Registry (ATSDR)	ATSDR, an agency within HHS, was created by the Superfund legislation to investigate and reduce the harmful effects of exposure to hazardous	No provisions.	Requires the Secretary to integrate ATSDR into plans for bioterrorism preparedness and response. Authorizes such sums as necessary for FY2002–

Topic	Current Law	S. 1765 Frist/Kennedy	H.R. 3448 Tauzin/Dingell
	substances on human health.		FY2006. for ATSDR's bioterrorism-related activities. [Section 137]
Federal Bioterrorism Web Site	No statutory provisions.	Recommends establishing a federal Web site on bioterrorism with links to state and local government sites. [Section 214]	No provisions.
Miscellaneous Provisions	No applicable provisions.	No provisions.	Requires the Secretary, in consultation with other federal agencies, to conduct a study of the ability of local public health entities to maintain communications during a public health emergency. [Section 111] Adds a new Section 319J to the PHS Act allowing the Secretary to provide supplies, equipment, or services instead of, or in conjunction with, grants awarded under Sections 319 through 3191, or Section 319K. [Section 112] Requires the Secretary to conduct a study of best practices in local emergency response and report to Congress within 180 days. [Section 114]
Medicare, Medicaid, and the State Children's Health Insurance Program (SCHIP)			
Emergency Waivers	Medicare covers medically necessary acute care and follow-up services (hospital, short-term nursing home care, physician services, home health and a variety of outpatient services) for	No provisions.	Authorizes the Secretary to temporarily waive conditions of participation and other certification requirements for any entity that furnishes health care items or services

Topic	Current Law	S. 1765 Frist/Kennedy	H.R. 3448 Tauzin/Dingell
	all persons age 65 and over, as well as certain disabled persons. Medicaid covers acute and long-term care services for low-income persons who are aged, blind, disabled, members of families with dependent children, and certain other pregnant women and children. The State Children's Health Insurance Program (SCHIP) covers uninsured children living in families with income above applicable Medicaid standards, typically up to or above 200% of the federal poverty level. In all three programs, providers must meet certain standards in order to participate and receive reimbursement for services rendered to program beneficiaries. For example, hospitals and other facilities must meet established conditions of participation, and laboratories must be certified under the Clinical Laboratories Improvement Act (CLIA). Physicians must be licensed to provide medical services in the state where medical care is rendered, and must follow established rules for obtaining prior approval to deliver certain types of services. Also, physicians must not refer patients to medical entities with which they have a financial		to Medicare, Medicaid, or SCHIP beneficiaries in an emergency area during a declared disaster or public health emergency. In addition, during such an emergency, authorizes the Secretary to waive: (i) participation, state licensing (as long as equivalent licensure from another state is held), and pre-approval requirements for physicians and other practitioners; (ii) sanctions for failing to meet requirements for emergency transfers between hospitals; and (iii) sanctions for physician self-referral. Requires the Secretary to provide Congress with a detailed written notice at least 2 days prior to exercising this waiver authority. Provides for the waiver authority to continue for 90 days. Permits the Secretary to extend the waiver period. Requires the Secretary, within 1 year after the end of the emergency, to provide Congress with an evaluation of the success of this approach and recommendations for improvements under this waiver authority. [Section 133]

Topic	Current Law	S. 1765 Frist/Kennedy	H.R. 3448 Tauzin/Dingell
	relationship. Other statutory provisions require hospitals to fully stabilize patients receiving emergency care prior to transfer to another medical facility.		
Regulation of Biological Agents and Toxins			
Use and Possession of Select Agents	The 1996 Antiterrorism and Effective Death Penalty Act (P.L. 104-132, Section 511) required the Secretary to establish a list of biological agents that could pose a severe threat to public health and safety, and establish safety procedures for transferring listed agents and toxins so as to protect public safety and prevent access by terrorists (see 42 C.F.R. 72).	Codifies and expands provisions of P.L. 104-132 in the PHS Act under a new Section 351A. Requires the Secretary to: (i) establish and, at least biennially, review and, if necessary, revise a list of biological agents and toxins that could pose a severe threat to public health and safety; (ii) establish safety procedures for transferring listed agents and toxins so as to protect public safety and prevent access by terrorists; (iii) establish standards and procedures for the possession and use of listed agents and toxins so as to protect public health and safety; and (iv) require registration for the possession, use, and transfer of listed agents and toxins and maintain a national database of the location of such agents and toxins. Requires the Secretary to establish security requirements for persons possessing, using, or transferring listed agents or toxins, as a condition of registration. Authorizes the Secretary to conduct compliance inspections. Authorizes the	Similar provisions to S. 1765, but with added security provisions: (i) requires the Secretary to consult with the Attorney General in establishing security requirements for persons possessing, using, or transferring listed agents or toxins; and (ii) requires the Secretary, in consultation with the Attorney General and other federal agencies, to establish a screening protocol to ensure that access to such agents and toxins is not permitted by certain specified types of individuals (e.g., those with criminal records, suspected terrorists, etc.). Requires the Secretary to coordinate regulations promulgated under these provisions with Dept. of Agriculture regulations governing use of biological agents in developing animal vaccines and treatments. Clarifies that the Secretary's new authorities do not limit existing authorities of the Secretary of Agriculture. Authorizes such sums as may be necessary for

Topic	Current Law	S. 1765 Frist/Kennedy	H.R. 3448 Tauzin/Dingell
		Secretary to establish exemptions from the requirements outlined in (ii) and (iii) above that are consistent with protecting public health and safety, including exemptions for the use of attenuated or inactive agents or toxins in research or for medical purposes. Exempts clinical labs presented with a listed agent or toxin for diagnosis, verification, or proficiency testing. Establishes civil penalties of up to $500,000 and criminal penalties of up to 5 years in prison for those in violation of the above requirements for the possession, use, and transfer of listed agents and toxins. Protects information collected under these regulations from mandatory disclosure under the Freedom of Information Act. Mandates a report to Congress within 1 year. Repeals current law. [Section 216]	FY2002, and each subsequent fiscal year, to upgrade security at HHS facilities that contain listed agents and toxins. [Section 201]
State and Local Preparedness and Response Capacity			
Bioterrorism Preparedness Grants to States and Local Public Health Agencies, and Health Care Facilities	PHS Act Section 319F(c) authorizes grants to states, localities, and health care facilities to increase their capacity to detect, diagnose, and respond to bioterrorist attacks, including training of personnel. [Note: For all activities under Section 319F, authorizes $215 million for FY2001, and such sums as	Amends PHS Act Section 319F(c) by replacing the existing grant program with block grants to states based on population, but with each state guaranteed a minimum level of funding. Requires states to develop a detailed bioterrorism preparedness plan to be eligible for funding. Authorizes $667	Amends PHS Act Section 319F(c) by expanding the existing grant authorization to permit the use of funds for community-wide planning activities, training, and purchasing or upgrading equipment, supplies, pharmaceuticals, and other countermeasures. Authorizes $455

Topic	Current Law	S. 1765 Frist/Kennedy	H.R. 3448 Tauzin/Dingell
	may be necessary for FY2002–FY2006.]	million for FY2002, and such sums as may be necessary for FY2003. [Section 301]	million for FY2002, and such sums as may be necessary for FY2003–FY2006. [Section 108, 151]
Core Capacity Grants to State and Local Public Health Agencies	PHS Act Section 319C authorizes grants to states and local governments, after they have completed a Section 319B evaluation, to address core public health capacity needs. Requires the Secretary to report to Congress on activities carried out under Sections 319A, 319B, and 319C by January 1, 2005. Authorizes $50 million for FY2001, and such sums as may be necessary for FY2002–FY2006.	Amends PHS Act Section 319C by authorizing $420 million for FY2002, and such sums as may be necessary for FY2003–FY2006. [Section 215]	Amends PHS Act Section 319C by expanding the existing grant authorization to permit the use of funds for purchasing or upgrading equipment, supplies, pharmaceuticals, and other countermeasures. Authorizes $455 million for FY2002, and such sums as may be necessary for FY2003–FY2006. [Section 109, 151]
Demonstration Grants	PHS Act Section 319G authorizes up to three demonstration grants for up to 5 years to states, localities, or non-profit organizations to carry out programs to improve biopathogen detection, develop plans for responding to bioterrorist attacks, and train response personnel. Requires a GAO report to Congress at the conclusion of the demonstration programs describing the capabilities of the grantees. Authorizes $6 million for FY2001, and such sums as may be necessary for FY2002–FY2006.	No provisions.	No provisions.

Topic	Current Law	S. 1765 Frist/Kennedy	H.R. 3448 Tauzin/Dingell
Grants to Hospitals	No applicable provisions.	Amends PHS Act Section 319F by establishing a grant program for hospitals and other medical centers to improve bioterrorism preparedness and response capacity. To be eligible, a hospital must form a consortium with a public health agency and a local government, and its grant proposal must be consistent with the state's bioterrorism preparedness plan. Requires the Secretary to develop and publish technical guidelines relating to equipment, training, treatment, capacity, and personnel. Authorizes $370 million for FY2002, and such sums as may be necessary for FY2003–FY2006. [Section 301, 311]	No provisions.
Grants to Address National Shortages of Specific Types of Health Professionals	No applicable provisions, although PHS Act Titles VII (Health Professionals Education) and VIII (Nursing Workforce Development) authorize federal support for training of health professionals for specific purposes.	No provisions.	Adds a new Section 319H to the PHS Act establishing a grant program to provide financial assistance for the education and training of individuals in any category of the health professions where there is a shortage that the Secretary determines should be alleviated to improve emergency readiness. Authorizes $40 million for FY2002, and such sums as may be necessary for FY2003–FY2006. [Section 106, 151]

Topic	Current Law	S. 1765 Frist/Kennedy	H.R. 3448 Tauzin/Dingell
Health Professional Volunteers	No applicable provisions.	No provisions.	Adds a new Section 3191 to the PHS Act requiring the Secretary to establish a national system to help verify the licenses, credentials, and hospital privileges of health professionals who volunteer to respond during public health emergencies. Authorizes $2 million for FY2002, and such sums as may be necessary for FY2003–FY2006. [Section 107]
State Public Emergency Announcements	The Stafford Act (42 U.S.C. 5121 et seq.) authorizes federal assistance when the President determines that a natural or man-made disaster has overwhelmed state and local resources. Stafford assistance is administered by the Federal Emergency Management Agency (FEMA).	Amends Section 613(b) of the Stafford Act by requiring states to include a plan for providing a coordinated public communications response in their submission for federal funds to help pay for state emergency preparedness personnel and administrative expenses. [Section 312]	Same provisions as S. 1765. [Section 135]
Countermeasures (Research, Development, and Production of New Vaccines, Drugs, and Technologies)			
Antitrust Exemption	The Clayton Act (15 U.S.C. 12 et seq.) is one of the federal antitrust laws that seek to promote fair competition and protect consumers and businesses from anti-competitive business practices. It enumerates specific practices that are anti-competitive and therefore forbidden.	Amends Section 2 of the Clayton Act to exempt from antitrust law meetings between the Secretary and parties involved in the development, manufacture, distribution, purchase and sale of new priority countermeasures against bioterrorism. Permits the Attorney General, in consultation with the Chairman of the Federal Trade	No provisions.

Topic	Current Law	S. 1765 Frist/Kennedy	H.R. 3448 Tauzin/Dingell
		Commission, to grant a limited antitrust exemption to agreements reached at such meetings. Limited exemptions expire after 3 years, but may be renewed. Terminates the Attorney General's authority to grant limited antitrust exemptions after 6 years. [Section 401]	
Smallpox Vaccine	No statutory provisions. In November 2001, HHS awarded a $428 million contact to Acambis, Inc. and Baxter International Inc. to produce 155 million doses of smallpox vaccine by the end of 2002. This is in addition to an earlier contract with Acambis to produce 54 million doses of the vaccine.	Adds new Section 2841 to the PHS Act requiring the Secretary to ensure adequate supplies of smallpox and other vaccines in the National Pharmaceutical Stockpile. Authorizes $509 million for FY2002, and such sums as may be necessary for FY2003–FY2006, to purchase smallpox vaccine. Adds a new Section 2842 to the PHS Act authorizing the Secretary to enter into long-term contracts with companies to purchase specific quantities of priority countermeasures at an agreed price. [Section 402]	Authorizes $509 million for FY2002, and such sums as may be necessary for FY2003–FY2006, to purchase smallpox vaccine. [Section 151]
Research and Development	PHS Act Section 319F requires the Secretary, in consultation with the interagency working group, to conduct research on the epidemiology and pathogenesis of biopathogens, diagnostic tests for biopathogens, and vaccines and other therapeutics.	Amends PHS Act Section 319F to: (i) make the genetic sequencing of biopathogens a priority at NIH; and (ii) expand research on the epidemiology and detection of biological agents and toxins, and the development of new vaccines and therapies. [Section 403, 404]	Amends PHS Act Section 319F to expand research on countermeasures, including the epidemiology and detection of biological agents and toxins, and the development of new vaccines and therapies. Defines a priority countermeasure as any drug, device, biologic, or diagnostic test to treat, identify, or prevent infection by

Topic	Current Law	S. 1765 Frist/Kennedy	H.R. 3448 Tauzin/Dingell
			a listed biological agent or toxin, or prevent harm from any other agent that may cause a pubic health emergency. Directs the Secretary to consider research collaboration with the VA. [Section 125]
FDA Approval of Drugs and Biologics	Under the Federal Food, Drug, and Cosmetic Act (FFDCA; 21 U.S.C. 301 et seq.), manufacturers of drugs and biologics (e.g., vaccines) must provide clinical trial data to demonstrate that their product is safe and effective, in order to obtain FDA marketing approval. The FFDCA provides for the designation of products as fast track to expedite the approval process.	Authorizes the Secretary to designate a priority countermeasure (i.e., drug or device) as a fast-track product for accelerated approval by the FDA. Permits a drug seeking FDA approval on the basis of animal data to be designated a fast-track product. Requires the FDA, within 30 days, to issue as a final rule the October 5, 1999 proposed rule permitting the use of animal data for approving new drugs and vaccines, when ethical issues preclude conducting clinical trials. [Section 405, 406]	Authorizes the Secretary to designate a priority countermeasure (i.e., drug or biologic) as a fast-track product for accelerated approval by the FDA but does not permit a drug seeking FDA approval on the basis of animal data to be designated a fast-track product. Requires the FDA, within 180 days, to issue as a final rule the October 5, 1999 proposed rule permitting the use of animal data for approving new drugs and vaccines, when ethical issues preclude conducting clinical trials. [Section 122, 123]
Security at Research and Production Facilities	No applicable provisions.	Adds a new Section 2843 to the PHS Act authorizing the Secretary, in consultation with the Secretary of Defense and the Attorney General, to provide technical or other assistance to enhance security at research and production facilities. Requires the Secretary to develop guidelines and best practices. [Section 402]	Adds a new Section 319K to the PHS Act authorizing the Secretary, in consultation with the Secretary of Defense and the Attorney General, to provide technical or other assistance to enhance security at research and production facilities. [Section 124]

Topic	Current Law	S. 1765 Frist/Kennedy	H.R. 3448 Tauzin/Dingell
Detection, Identification, Diagnosis, and Surveillance Technologies	No applicable provisions.	No provisions.	Requires the Secretary to evaluate and prioritize new and emerging technologies for responding to a bioterrorism attack or other public health emergency. Requires the Secretary to report to Congress within 180 days on those technologies whose development should be accelerated. [Section 126] Requires the Secretary of Energy and the Administrator of the National Nuclear Safety Administration, in coordination with the interagency working group, to expand research on the rapid detection and identification of biopathogens. Authorizes such sums as may be necessary for FY2002–FY2006. [Section 136]
Potassium Iodide	No applicable provisions.	No provisions.	Requires the Secretary to make potassium iodide available from the national pharmaceutical stockpile to states and local governments that submit a plan for local stockpile and distribution to the population within 20 miles of a nuclear power plant. Requires the Secretary, within 6 months, to provide Congress with a progress report. [Section 127]

Topic	Current Law	S. 1765 Frist/Kennedy	H.R. 3448 Tauzin/Dingell
Antimicrobial Resistance			
Combating Antimicrobial Resistance	PHS Act 319E requires the Secretary to establish an Antimicrobial Resistance Task Force to coordinate federal programs on antimicrobial resistance and to work on surveillance plans and information systems for detection and control of drug-resistant pathogens. Authorizes research and development initiatives for new antimicrobial drugs and diagnostics. Directs the Secretary to conduct a nationwide campaign to educate the public and health care professionals about the appropriate use of antibiotics. Authorizes grants for public health agencies to combat antimicrobial resistance. Authorizes demonstration grants for hospitals, clinics, and other entities to promote the judicious use of antibiotics and to control the spread of resistant infections. Authorizes $40 million for FY2001, and such sums as may be necessary for FY2002–FY2006.	No provisions.	Amends PHS Act Section 319E to authorize additional research on priority pathogens. Authorizes $25 million for FY2002 and for FY2003, and such sums as may be necessary for FY2004–FY2006. [Section 110, 151]
Drug and Device Supply Safety and Security			
Drug and Device Importation	FFDCA Section 510(i) requires foreign drug and device manufacturers that import into the United States to register with the Secretary their name, place of	No provisions.	Amends Section 510(i) of the FFDCA by mandating annual registration of foreign manufacturers engaged in the import of drugs and devices into the

Topic	Current Law	S. 1765 Frist/Kennedy	H.R. 3448 Tauzin/Dingell
	business, and the name of their U.S. agent. Section 801 governs the import and export of food, drugs, devices, and other items, and specifies the circumstances under which imported articles are inspected, detained, or refused entry into the United States.		United States. Requires registration to include the name of each importer and carrier used by the manufacturer. Amends Section 801 so that an imported drug or device may be refused entry if the importer fails to give the Secretary a statement identifying each foreign establishment that, under the law, must also be registered. [Section 311]
Import Components Intended for Export	FFDCA Section 301 is the prohibited acts and penalties section of the statute. Section 801 governs the import and export of food, drugs, devices, and other items, and specifies the circumstances under which imported articles are inspected, detained, or refused entry into the United States.	No provisions.	Amends Section 801 of the FFDCA mandating a chain-of-possession identification and a customs bond for firms seeking to import components of drugs, devices, food additives, color additives, or dietary supplements for further processing and export. Requires certificates of analysis for components containing any chemical or biological substance intended for export. Permits the Secretary to exclude from importation any article for which there is credible evidence or information indicating that the article presents a serious health threat or death to humans or animals. Amends Section 301 making it illegal to knowingly submit false statements, certificates, records, or reports required under Section 801, as

Topic	Current Law	S. 1765 Frist/Kennedy	H.R. 3448 Tauzin/Dingell
			amended. [Section 312]
Food Supply Safety and Security			
Strategic Plan for Food Safety and Security	Executive Order 13100 created the President's Council on Food Safety, headed by the Secretaries of Agriculture and Health and Human Services, the Administrator of the Environmental Protection Agency, and the Assistant to the President for Science and Technology. On January 18, 2001, the Council published a strategic plan for food safety that contained recommendations on making statutory changes to unify federal food safety regulations.	Requires the Council, along with the Secretaries of Commerce and Transportation, and in consultation with states, the food industry, and consumer and producer groups, to develop a crisis communications and education strategy for bioterrorist threats to the food supply that includes threat assessments, response and notification procedures, and public risk communication plans. Authorizes $500,000 for FY2002, and such sums as may be necessary in each subsequent fiscal year, to implement the strategy. [Section 511]	No provisions.
U.S. Department of Agriculture (USDA) Activities	USDA's Food Safety and Inspection Service (FSIS) inspects meat, poultry, and processed egg products sold for human consumption for safety, wholesomeness, and proper labeling. The Animal and Plant Inspection Service (APHIS) inspects cargo and passengers at U.S. ports for animal and plant pests, quarantines some of these products, and responds to animal disease outbreaks. The Agricultural Research Service (ARS) conducts research on animal diseases and food	Authorizes $15 million for enhanced FSIS inspections domestically and internationally and collaboration with other federal agencies; $30 million for APHIS for increased inspections, cooperative agreements with state and private veterinarians, and an automated, integrated, interagency emergency warning, response, and record-keeping system; and $180 million for upgrading biosecurity at ARS labs in New York and Iowa. Authorizes the Secretary of Agriculture to use $20 million in	No provisions.

Topic	Current Law	S. 1765 Frist/Kennedy	H.R. 3448 Tauzin/Dingell
	safety to support other USDA regulatory responsibilities.	FY2002 to award up to $45,000 each to land grant universities to establish security at facilities, inventory hazardous toxins, develop a screening protocol for access to facilities, and develop industry-on-farm education program. Authorizes a total of $245 million for FY2002 for USDA biosecurity efforts and such sums as necessary for each fiscal year thereafter. [Section 512, 513, 515, 527]	
HHS and FDA Biosecurity	FFDCA Chapter IV prohibits the entry into interstate commerce of adulterated or misbranded foods. FDA monitors through inspections whether food manufacturers adhere to their legal responsibility to produce food that is not defective, unsafe, filthy, or produced under unsanitary conditions.	Requires the Secretary of HHS to secure existing facilities where potential animal or plant pathogens are housed and researched. Authorizes $59 million to expand FDA's inspections and collaboration with other federal, state, and tribal agencies. Authorizes $500,000 for the Secretary to develop best practices for biosecurity for use by food manufacturers, processors, and distributors. Authorizes a total of $59.5 million for FY2002 for HHS agencies and such sums as may be necessary for each fiscal year thereafter. [Section 514,516,518]	Authorizes a total of $100 million for the Secretary of HHS to increase inspections for the detection of intentional adulteration of imported food; to give high priority to improving FDA's information management systems; to develop tests and sampling methods to rapidly detect intentionally adulterated food; and to complete an assessment of threats to food posed by intentional adulteration and report its findings on these protective activities to Congress. [Section 301]
Food Detention	FFDCA Section 304 allows for the seizure of food in interstate commerce under restricted circumstances.	Amends FFDCA Section 304 to authorize the detention of food for 20 days, and if needed for 30 days, if an officer or qualified employee of FDA	Similar to provisions in S. 1765, except that it limits detention approval authority to the Secretary or the Secretary's designee. It also does not

Topic	Current Law	S. 1765 Frist/Kennedy	H.R. 3448 Tauzin/Dingell
		has credible evidence (and the Secretary approves) showing the food violates the FFDCA and presents a threat of serious adverse health consequences or death to humans or animals. The detained food must be secured, and the responsible person can file an appeal within 15 days with expedited procedures for perishable foods. Adds a new definition to FFDCA Section 310 prohibiting removal of product or mark or label from the detained product. [Section 531]	set a time limit on the appeal, but does require that FDA make a final decision within 72 hours on the appeal. Authorizes the Secretary to request the Treasury Secretary to temporarily hold imported food at a port for 24 hours, if FDA has credible evidence indicating that the food presents a threat, to allow FDA to determine whether to detain it. Requires that the Secretary notify the state in which the involved port is located. [Section 302]
Debarment for Food Imports	FFDCA Section 306 gives the Secretary of HHS authority to debar, temporarily deny approval, or suspend the rights of individuals who have been convicted of a felony to submit an application for approval of a drug.	Amends FFDCA Section 306 to debar from importing foods any person who is convicted of a felony related to the importation of food or who repeatedly imports, or knows, or should have known, that the imported food that was adulterated or misbranded. Amends FFDCA Section 402 to include in the definition of "adulterated food" any food imported by debarred persons. [Section 532]	Similar provisions. [Section 303]
Maintenance and Inspection of Records	FFDCA Section 704 authorizes FDA to conduct factory inspections. Currently, FDA inspectors have access to company records but can only request access to copy, and verify records for restricted medical devices, prescription	Add a new Section 414 to the FFDCA allowing the Secretary, if a food is believed to be adulterated or misbranded and presents a threat of serious adverse health consequences or death to humans or animals, to have access to and to copy	Similar provisions to S. 1765, but includes language that requires the Secretary to put into effect procedures to prevent unauthorized disclosure of any trade secrets or confidential information. Also provides authority

Topic	Current Law	S. 1765 Frist/Kennedy	H.R. 3448 Tauzin/Dingell
	drugs, not for foods. Inspectors may not require that records be kept nor do officials have authority to copy records found during inspections.	all records related to the food. Excludes restaurants and farms, and has reduced requirements for small businesses (less than 50 employees.) Requires records to be kept for 2 years so food can be investigated. Excludes records on USDA-regulated foods (meat, poultry, and egg products), and on trade secrets and/or confidential information on recipes, and financial, pricing, personnel, research, and sales data. Amends FFDCA Section 704 to add a clause to allow the inspection of all records and other information described in the new Section 414. Requires final rules to be issued on record keeping within 18 months. [Section 533]	to the Secretary to take into account the size of the business when imposing any record keeping requirements. Does not impose a time limit for promulgation of rules. [Section 304]
Registration of Food Facilities	Currently, only States have records of food processing, packing and holding facilities. The federal government must ask the states for this information.	Creates a new Section 415 in the FFDCA requiring all facilities, domestic and foreign, that manufacture, process, and handle food to register with the Secretary all the identities (brand names) under which business is conducted, addresses of the facilities, and general food categories. Foreign registrations must name a U.S. agent. Requires the Secretary to give each facility a number and keep the list of registered facilities up to date. Exempts certain retail stores and farms from registration	Similar provisions to S. 1765, but applies requirements to facilities that manufacture, process, pack or hold food (excludes farms.) Adds that the Secretary may provide for and encourage the use of electronic submissions to register as long as there are authorization protocols used to identify the registrant and validate the data. Adds that the Secretary must within 60 days identify facilities required to register, and, as S. 1765, enforce the registration within 180

Topic	Current Law	S. 1765 Frist/Kennedy	H.R. 3448 Tauzin/Dingell
		requirements. Registration does not imply a license. Requirements for registration would take effect 180 days after enactment. Amends Section 403 to prohibit interstate commerce of food from unregistered facilities. [Section 534]	days of the Act's enactment. Exempts only retail establishments from registration requirements. Specifies that registration requirements would not apply to food products regulated by USDA. [Section 305]
Prior Notice of Imported Food Shipments	Under FFDCA Section 801, a food that (i) is found to be manufactured, processed, or packed under unsanitary conditions, (ii) is forbidden or restricted in the producing country or from where it was exported, or (iii) is adulterated or misbranded at the border, can have its admission deferred while the food is reconditioned, relabeled or destroyed.	Amends FFDCA Section 801 to require a producer, manufacturer, or shipper of imported food, at least 4 hours before it is imported, to document its identity, country of origin, and quantity imported to FDA and the U.S. Customs or the import can be refused entry. Exempts all USDA-regulated foods (meat, poultry, and egg products.) Prohibits knowingly making a false statement in the import documentation. [Section 535]	Similar provisions to S. 1765, except the advance period for submission of documentation is to be not less than 24 hours nor more than 72 hours before importation of the food. The required information includes a description of the food, the identity of the manufacturer and shipper, if possible the grower, the country of origin of the food, the country from which the article is shipped, and the anticipated U.S. port of entry. Without a notice, the food will be refused admission or held until the required information is provided and a determination that the food is not a serious health threat to humans or animals. The Secretary can ask for more information. This provision excludes USDA regulated products. [Section 306]

Topic	Current Law	S. 1765 Frist/Kennedy	H.R. 3448 Tauzin/Dingell
Mark Articles Refused Admission	The FFDCA Section 403 defines misbranded foods as food whose labeling or advertising is false or misleading. Section 801(a) gives the Secretary the general authority to refuse imports deemed adulterated or misbranded.	Amends both Sections 403 and 801(a) definitions of misbranded food to include food that has been refused admission to the United States and not destroyed and which presents a threat of serious adverse health consequences or death, unless the packaging is clearly and conspicuously labeled: *United States: Refused Entry* at the expense of the food's owner until the food is brought into compliance. [Section 536]	Similar provisions to S. 1765. [Section 307]
Authority to Commission Other Federal Officials to Conduct Inspections	The FFDCA Section 702 states that the Secretary is authorized to conduct food inspections (examinations and investigations) through officers and employees of HHS, or any health, food, or drug officer of a state that has been duly commissioned by the Secretary as an officer of the Department.	Amends FFDCA Section 702 to provide the authority to commission qualified federal officials from other departments or agencies to conduct inspections. This can only happen if there are no current laws restricting the use of a department or agency officers, employees, or funds. [Section 537]	No provisions.
Prohibition against Port Shopping	The FFDCA Section 402 defines "adulterated" food as any food that bears or contains any poisonous or deleterious substance that may render it injurious to health.	Amends FFDCA Section 402 to require that an importer offering food that has been refused admission prove at his own expense that the food is in compliance with the applicable requirements of the Act. [Section 538]	Similar provisions to S. 1765 except that importer, at his own expense, must prove that the article is not adulterated, as determined by the Secretary. [Section 308]
Grants to States for Inspections	The FFDCA Section 702 states that the Secretary is authorized to conduct food inspections (examinations and investigations) through officers and	Creates a new Section 910 in the FFDCA authorizing $10 million for FY2002, and such sums as may be necessary for subsequent fiscal years, to	Creates a new Section 909 in the FFDCA authorizing grants to states and territories to conduct food safety examinations, inspections, and

Topic	Current Law	S. 1765 Frist/Kennedy	H.R. 3448 Tauzin/Dingell
	employees of HHS, or any health, food, or drug officer of a state that has been duly commissioned by the Secretary as an officer of the Department.	provide grants to states to increase food safety examinations, inspections and investigations under FFDCA Section 702. [Section 539]	investigations under Section 702, like S. 1765, but does not specify an amount. Also, allows grants to states to assist in costs when responding to adulterated food that might injure public health. [Section 310]
Notices to States Regarding Imported Food	No provisions.	No provisions.	Requires that the Secretary notify the state that holds the food when there is credible evidence that it presents a threat of serious adverse health consequences or death to humans or animals. [Section 309]
Rule of Construction	USDA regulates meat under the Federal Meat Inspection Act (21 U.S.C. 601 et seq.), poultry under the Poultry Products Inspection Act (21 U.S.C. 451 et seq.), and processed egg products under the Egg Products Inspection Act (21 U.S.C. 1031 et seq.)	Prohibits FDA from regulating any food under USDA's jurisdiction. [Section 540]	No provisions.
Food Safety Grants	FoodNet, established in 1995 by USDA and FDA, tracks the incidence of illnesses caused by nine pathogens in nine geographic areas across the United States. PulseNet compares genetic patterns of bacteria isolated from patients with foodborne illness and/or contaminated food.	Amends PHS Act Title III to authorize $19.5 million for FY2002 in grants to states to expand the number participating in FoodNet and PulseNet and other surveillance networks and to maintain technical and laboratory capacity. [Section 541]	No provisions.
Surveillance of Animal and Human	CDC has more than 20 surveillance programs that monitor outbreaks of	Amends PHS Act Title III to authorize FDA, CDC, and USDA to develop and	No provisions.

Topic	Current Law	S. 1765 Frist/Kennedy	H.R. 3448 Tauzin/Dingell
Health	food borne illness caused by specific pathogens.	implement a plan for coordinating surveillance for zoonotic and human diseases. [Section 541]	
Agricultural Bioterrorism Research and Development	Current research programs are in place in the Agricultural Research Service (ARS) and the Cooperative Research Service Education and Extension Service (CSREES).	Expands, with an authorization of $190 million for FY2002 and such sums as may be necessary for subsequent fiscal years, the programs of USDA's agencies ARS and CSREES to protect the food supply and expand links with the intelligence community and international organizations. [Section 542]	No provisions.
Drinking Water Security and Safety			
Vulnerability Assessments and Emergency Response Plans	PHS Act Title XIV, the Safe Drinking Water Act (SDWA), authorizes federal regulation of public water systems (including community water systems), particularly through a program that regulates contaminants in public water supplies. The Act defines a community water system as a public water system that serves at least 15 service connections served by year-round residents or that regularly serves at least 25 year-round residents. The SDWA is administered and enforced by the Environmental Protection Agency (EPA).	No provisions.	Adds a new Section 1433 to the SDWA to require each community water system serving more than 3,300 individuals to conduct a vulnerability assessment. Requires EPA, not later than March 1, 2002, to provide information to community water systems concerning probable threats. Establishes deadlines for systems to certify to EPA that they have conducted vulnerability assessments. Requires each community water system serving more than 3,300 individuals to prepare or revise an emergency response plan incorporating the results of the vulnerability assessment. Systems

Topic	Current Law	S. 1765 Frist/Kennedy	H.R. 3448 Tauzin/Dingell
			must certify to EPA, no later than 6 months after completing an assessment, that they have completed response plans. Directs EPA to provide guidance to community water systems serving fewer than 3,300 individuals on conducting vulnerability assessments, preparing emergency response plans, and addressing threats from terrorist attacks or other actions intended to disrupt the provision of safe drinking water. Authorizes $120 million for FY2002, and such sums as may be necessary for FY2003 and FY2004, to provide financial assistance to community water systems to conduct assessments and prepare response plans, and for expenses and contracts to address basic security enhancements and significant threats. [Section 401(1)]
Review of Methods to Prevent, Detect, and Respond to the Intentional Introduction of Contaminants into Community Water Supplies	No statutory provisions.	No provisions.	Adds new SDWA Section 1434 directing the EPA Administrator, in consultation with CDC, and after consultation with other federal departments and state and local governments, to review current and future methods to prevent, detect and respond to the intentional introduction

Topic	Current Law	S. 1765 Frist/Kennedy	H.R. 3448 Tauzin/Dingell
			of chemical, biological or radiological contaminants into community water systems and their source waters. Provides that funding is authorized under Section 1435. [Section 401(1)]
Supply Disruption: Prevention, Detection and Response	No statutory provisions.	No provisions.	Adds new SDWA Section 1435 directing the EPA Administrator, in coordination with appropriate federal departments and agencies, to review methods and means by which terrorists or others could disrupt the supply of safe drinking water or take actions that render water unsafe, including methods and means by which water systems could be destroyed, impaired, or made subject to cross-contamination. EPA must also review methods and means by which systems could be reasonably protected from attacks, and by which alternative drinking water supplies could be provided if a water system was destroyed, impaired or contaminated. Authorizes $15 million for FY2002, and such sums as may be necessary for FY2003 and FY2004 to carry out Sections 1434 and 1435. [Section 401(1)]
Enforceable Requirements	SDWA Section 1414(i)(1) identifies the sections of SDWA for which the Act's	No provisions.	Amends SDWA Section 1414(i)(1) to include new Section 1433, requiring

Topic	**Current Law**	**S. 1765 Frist/Kennedy**	**H.R. 3448 Tauzin/Dingell**
	enforcement authorities apply.		community water systems to conduct vulnerability assessments and to prepare emergency response plans, as an applicable and enforceable requirement under the Act. [Section 401(2)]
Emergency Powers	SDWA Section 1431 grants the EPA Administrator emergency powers to take such actions as deemed necessary to protect persons served by a public water system upon receipt of information that a contaminant which is present in or is likely to enter a public water system or groundwater source may present an imminent and substantial endangerment to health of those persons.	No provisions.	Amends SDWA Section 1431 to specify that EPA's emergency powers include the authority to act when there is a threatened or potential terrorist attack or other intentional act to disrupt the provision of safe drinking water or to impact the safety of a community's drinking water supply. [Section 401(3)]
Penalties for Tampering with Public Water Systems	SDWA Section 1432 authorizes criminal and civil penalties for persons who tamper, attempt to tamper, or threaten to tamper with public water supplies.	No provisions.	Amends SDWA Section 1432 to increase criminal and civil penalties for tampering, attempting to tamper, or making threats to tamper with public water supplies. [Section 401(4)]
Technical Assistance	SDWA Section 1442(b) authorizes EPA to provide technical assistance and to make grants to states and public water systems to assist in responding to and alleviating emergency situations.	No provisions.	Amends SDWA Section 1442(d) to authorize appropriations to carry out Section 1442(b) of not more than $35 million for FY2002, and such sums as may be necessary for each fiscal year thereafter. [Section 401(5)]

APPENDIX A. HHS BIOTERRORISM FUNDING

FY1999–FY2001 Bioterrorism Initiative

HHS launched its bioterrorism initiative in FY1999. The initiative has six strategic goals: prevention of bioterrorism; infectious disease surveillance; medical and public health readiness for mass casualty events; the National Pharmaceutical Stockpile (NPS); research and development of new drugs and vaccines; and information technology infrastructure. Funding for these activities in the first 3 years (i.e., FY1999–FY2001) totaled about $730 million. CDC used the lion's share of those funds to begin the process of improving the bioterrorism preparedness and response capacity of state and local health departments. The agency awarded grants to state and major metropolitan health departments to support preparedness planning and readiness assessment; increase laboratory capacity for biological and chemical agents; and create the Health Alert Network, a nationwide, secure electronic communications network for state and local health departments. CDC has also used some of the funds to upgrade its own facilities and laboratory capacity and to establish and manage the NPS. In addition, HHS's Office of Emergency Preparedness (OEP) has expanded the National Disaster Medical System (see **Table 1**) and awarded grants to strengthen emergency medical response systems in metropolitan areas.

FY2002 FUNDING

For FY2002, Congress appropriated $3 billion to HHS to improve bioterrorism preparedness at the federal, state, and local levels. Bioterrorism funding was included in both the FY2002 Labor-HHS-Education appropriations bill and the anti-terrorism emergency-spending package.

Labor-HHS-Education Appropriations

The FY2002 Labor-HHS-Education appropriations act (P.L. 107-116, H.R. 3061) included $243 million for the bioterrorism initiative: $182 million for CDC and $61 million for OEP.

Emergency Supplemental Appropriations

Congress passed a $40 billion emergency supplemental appropriations bill (P.L. 107-38, H.R. 2888) within days of the September 11 attacks to provide aid to the victims, repair damaged public facilities and transportation systems, expand law enforcement activities, and strengthen counter-terrorism capabilities. The first $10 billion was available immediately for allocation by the President. An additional $10 billion was available 15 days after the President notified Congress about how he would distribute the funds. In a series of notifications beginning on September 21, 2001, the Administration allocated all but $327 million of the first $20 billion before the 15-day prior notification period expired on

November 25. Those allocations included $121 million for HHS to provide emergency assistance for health care and social services in the New York and Washington, DC, metropolitan areas.[2]

The second $20 billion was made subject to the appropriations process and was included as an amendment to the FY2002 Defense Department appropriations bill (P.L. 107-117, H.R. 3338). As enacted, H.R. 3338 provides HHS a total of $2.8 billion for bioterrorism-related activities. The appropriations act allocates that funding under several broad categories, including $593 million for the NPS, $512 million to purchase smallpox vaccine, $865 million for state and local health departments, $135 million to upgrade hospital capacity, $100 million to upgrade CDC's facilities and capacity, $155 for NIH research and lab construction, and $151 for FDA lab security, vaccine approval, and food safety. The act also provides $140 million to reimburse Medicare, Medicaid, and other health care providers for expenses or lost revenues attributable to the September 11 attacks.

While lawmakers work towards final passage of new bioterrorism authorizing legislation, CDC and the Health Resources and Services Administration (HRSA) have awarded a total of $1 billion in FY2002 funds to upgrade state and local health departments and improve hospital preparedness and response capacity. See Appendix B for more information on these grant programs.

FY2003 Budget Request

The President's FY2003 budget would provide a total of $4.3 billion for HHS's bioterrorism preparedness programs and activities. The budget request includes funds for strengthening the federal medical and public health response capacity, upgrading CDC's facilities, improving state and local public health preparedness, developing vaccines and maintaining the National Pharmaceutical Stockpile, preparing the nation's hospitals, expanding FDA's regulatory oversight of drugs and biologics, and securing facilities to conduct critical scientific work. **Table 2** summarizes HHS's bioterrorism funding in FY2001, FY2002, and the FY2003 budget request.

Note that the table does not include the funding provided for recovery and relief efforts in response to the September 11 attacks (e.g., $121 million in emergency assistance to New York and Washington, DC, and $140 million to reimburse health care providers).

[2] The funds were used to provide emergency grants to health care providers, community health centers, and mental health and substance abuse centers, and to provide services for the disabled, home-delivered meals, and transportation for senior citizens in affected areas.

Table 2. HHS Bioterrorism Funding ($ millions)

Agency and Program	FY2001 Actual	FY2002 Enacted	FY2003 Request
Centers for Disease Control and Prevention (CDC)			
State and local public health preparedness	67	940	940
CDC capacity	22	116	144
National Pharmaceutical Stockpile	51	645	300
Smallpox vaccine procurement	0	512	100
Physical security and facilities	3	46	120
Other[a]	39	39	33
Subtotal, CDC	**$181**	**$2,298**	**$1,637**
Health Resources and Services Admin. (HRSA)			
Hospital preparedness and infrastructure	0	135	518
Other[b]	0	0	100
Subtotal, HRSA	**$0**	**$135**	**$618**
Food and Drug Administration (FDA)			
Food safety	1	98	98
Vaccine and drug approval	6	47	54
Physical security	2	13	7
Subtotal, FDA	**$8**	**$158**	**$159**
National Institutes of Health (NIH)			
Research	53	183	977
Physical security and facilities	0	92	521
Anthrax vaccine procurement	0	0	250
Subtotal, NIH	**$53**	**$274**	**$1,748**
Office of the Secretary (OS)			
Office of Emergency Preparedness[c]	33	76	117
Office of Public Health Preparedness	30	41	33
Subtotal, OS	**$63**	**$117**	**$150**
Substance Abuse & Mental Health Services Admin.	0	0	10
TOTAL, HHS Bioterrorism	**$305**	**$2,982**	**$4,322**

Source: Dept. Health and Human Services FY2003 Budget Request

Note: Columns may not add due to rounding.

[a] Includes funding for anthrax vaccine evaluation and research, and national planning.

[b] Includes funding for poison control centers, medical curricula, and addressing children's needs.

[c] Includes funding for the National Disaster Medical System (NDMS), the Metropolitan Medical Response Systems (MMRS) program, and HHS cybersecurity.

APPENDIX B. CDC AND HRSA BIOTERRORISM PREPAREDNESS GRANT PROGRAMS

For FY2002, Congress provided $940 million to CDC to upgrade state and local public health departments and $135 million to HRSA to increase hospital preparedness (see **Table 2**).

State and Local Public Health Department Preparedness

CDC established a cooperative agreement program (pursuant to authority in PHS Act Sections 319B, 319C, and 319F) to improve the preparedness of state and local public health departments to respond to bioterrorism, infectious disease outbreaks, and other public health threats and emergencies. On February 19, 2002, using a population-based allocation formula, CDC awarded $918 million in grants to the health departments of all 50 states, Washington DC, the five territories, and the nation's three largest cities (New York, Chicago, and Los Angeles County). While 20% of the award is available for immediate use, the remaining 80% is contingent on the approval of a state work plan to be submitted to CDC no later than April 15, 2002. According to the agency's guidance documents, work plans must describe the activities to be undertaken to develop and expand critical capacities in the following areas: preparedness planning and readiness assessment; surveillance and epidemiology; laboratory capacity; communications and information technology; and education and training. For more information on CDC's grant program, go to [http://www.bt.cdc.gov/Planning/CoopAgreementAward/index.asp].

Hospital Preparedness

HRSA's cooperative agreement program provides grants to improve the capacity of hospitals and other health care facilities to care for the victims of bioterrorism, natural infectious disease outbreaks, and other public health emergencies. The agency has awarded $125 million to the same entities that received CDC funding, using a similar population-based allocation formula. As with the CDC grants, the funds are being released in two phases. Phase one funding (20% of the total award) is subject to an application filed no later than Feb. 25, 2002. Phase two funding (80% of the total award) is contingent on an approved work plan due no later than April 15, 2002. Grantees are required to provide at least 80% of the phase two funds to hospitals. For more information on HRSA's hospital preparedness grant program, go to [http://www.hrsa.gov/bioterrorism.htm].

Coordination and Review of State Work Plans

DHHS has encouraged states to develop their public health and hospital preparedness plans in tandem. In an effort to ensure that the CDC and HRSA funds are used in a coordinated manner, grantees are required to submit both work plans to their governor (or mayor in the case of the municipalities) for approval. The governor (or mayor) is then required to transmit a letter of endorsement to the department. To date, HRSA has received 47 state work plans and granted extensions to three states. Montana and Utah have each received a one-month extension (until May 15), and Texas has been granted an extension until July 1. CDC has received 48 state work plans and granted one-month extensions to Montana and Utah. All four municipalities (i.e., Washington DC, New York City, Chicago, and Los Angeles County) have submitted their work plans to CDC and HRSA. The department's goal is to release all the grant funds to each state and municipality within 30 days of receipt of both work plans and the letter of endorsement from the governor (or mayor). For a table showing the amount of CDC and HRSA funding each state, territory, and municipality has received, go to [http://www.hhs.gov/news/press/2002pres/states.html].

Appendix C. Bioterrorism-Related Hearings (107TH Congress)

Senate Appropriations Subcommittee on Labor, HHS, and Education

- October 3, 2001 Bioterrorism: Public health preparedness and response
- October 23, 2001 Public health response to anthrax attack
- November 2, 2001 Smallpox: Public health preparedness and response
- November 29, 2001 Funding for bioterrorism preparedness

Senate Appropriations Subcommittee on VA-HUD and Independent Agencies

- November 28, 2001 Anthrax decontamination

Senate Armed Services Subcommittee on Emerging Threats and Capabilities

- October 25, 2001 Bioterrorism and the Dark Winter exercise

Senate Commerce, Science and Transportation Committee

- February 5, 2002 Bioterrorism: Countermeasures R&D (Subcommittee on Science, Technology, and Space)

Senate Environment and Public Works Committee

- December 4, 2001 Anthrax decontamination

Senate Foreign Relations Committee

- September 5, 2001 Bioterrorism threat and the spread of infectious diseases

Senate Governmental Affairs Committee

- July 23, 2001 Bioterrorism: FEMA's role and public health preparedness (Subcommittee on National Security, Proliferation and Federal Services)
- October 17, 2001 Bioterrorism: Federal agency preparedness
- October 30-31, 2001 Anthrax in the mail: Protecting postal workers and the public
- April 18, 2002 Public health preparedness

Senate Health, Education, Labor, and Pensions Committee

- September 26, 2001 Psychological trauma of terrorism
- October 9, 2001 Bioterrorism: Public health preparedness and response
- November 2, 2001 Kids and terrorism (Subcommittee on Children and Families)

Senate Judiciary Committee

- November 6, 2001 Law enforcement and the domestic bioterrorism threat (Subcommittee on Technology, Terrorism and Government Information)

House Appropriations Subcommittee on Labor, HHS, and Education

- May 1, 2002 HHS bioterrorism preparedness

House Energy and Commerce Committee

- October 10, 2001 Bioterrorism preparedness and response (Subcommittee on Oversight and Investigations)
- November 1, 2001 Public health early-warning surveillance systems (Subcommittee on Oversight and Investigations)
- November 7, 2001 Physical security and NIH and CDC facilities (Subcommittee on Oversight and Investigations)
- November 15, 2001 Bioterrorism: Public health preparedness and response

House Government Reform Committee

- May 1, 2001 Management of medical stockpiles (Subcommittee on National Security, Veterans Affairs and International Relations)

- July 23, 2001 Federal response to a bioterrorism attack: Dark Winter (Subcommittee on National Security, Veterans Affairs and International Relations)
- October 5, 2001 Bioterrorism: Federal, state, and local preparedness (Subcommittee on Government Efficiency, Financial Management and Intergovernmental Relations)
- October 12, 2001 Assessing the threat of bioterrorism (Subcommittee on National Security, Veterans Affairs and International Relations)
- October 23, 2001 Vaccine research and development (Subcommittee on National Security, Veterans Affairs and International Relations)
- October 30, 2001 Anthrax and postal worker safety
- November 7, 2001 DOD medical readiness for chemical and biological warfare (Subcommittee on National Security, Veterans Affairs and International Relations)
- November 14, 2001 Medical care for bioterrorism victims
- November 29, 2001 Risk communication: National security and public health (Subcommittee on National Security, Veterans Affairs and International Relations)
- December 14, 2001 Bioterrorism response: Information sharing between local, state, and federal governments (Subcommittee on Technology and Procurement Policy)
- February 28, 2002 Anthrax antitoxin research
- March 1, 2002 Federal, state, and local response to biological and chemical attack (Subcommittee on Government Efficiency, Financial Management and Intergovernmental Relations)
- March 21, 2002 Combating terrorism (Subcommittee on National Security, Veterans Affairs and International Relations)

House International Relations Committee

- December 5, 2001 Bioterrorism and potential sources of anthrax

House Science Committee

- November 8, 2001 Anthrax decontamination
- December 5, 2001 Bioterrorism: Federal preparedness and response

House Veterans' Affairs Committee

- April 10, 2002 Bioterrorism legislation (H.R. 3253, H.R. 3254)

Appendix D. Bioterrorism-Related Web Sites

Department of Health and Human Services

- Information on public health preparedness [http://www.hhs.gov/hottopics/healing]
- DHHS Office of Emergency Preparedness [http://www.oep.dhhs.gov]

- DHHS Office of Public Health Preparedness [http://www.hhs.gov/ophp]
- Metropolitan Medical Response Systems [http://www.mmrs.hhs.gov]
- National Pharmaceutical Stockpile Program [http://www.cdc.gov/nceh/nps]
- Centers for Disease Control and Prevention [http://www.bt.cdc.gov]
- Health Resources and Services Admin. [http://www.hrsa.gov/bioterrorism.htm]
- Food and Drug Administration [http://www.fda.gov/oc/opacom/hottopics/bioterrorism.html]
- National Institutes of Health [http://www.niaid.nih.gov/publications/bioterrorism.htm]
- National Library of Medicine [http://www.nlm.nih.gov/medlineplus/biologicalandchemicalweapons.html]

Department of Defense

- U.S. Army Medical Research Institute of Infectious Diseases [http://www.usamriid.army.mil]
- DOD Anthrax Vaccine Immunization Program [http://www.anthrax.osd.mil]
- Nuclear, Biological, Chemical Medical Reference Site [http://www.nbc-med.org/others]

State and Local Health Departments

Many health departments have included information on bioterrorism and public health preparedness on their Web sites. For links to state and local health departments, go to [http://www.apha.org/public_health/state.htm].

Professional Associations

- American College of Emergency Physicians [http://www.acep.org/1,4634,0.html]
- American College of Physicians [http://www.acponline.org/bioterro]
- American Hospital Association [http://www.aha.org/Emergency/EmIndex.asp]
- American Medical Association [http://www.ama-assn.org/ama/pub/category/6671.html]
- American Society for Microbiology [http://www.asm.org/pcsrc/bioprep.htm]
- Association for Professionals in Infection Control and Epidemiology [http://www.apic.org/bioterror]
- Association of State and Territorial Health Officials [http://www.astho.org/infectious/emerging.html]
- Council of State and Territorial Epidemiologists [http://www.cste.org]
- Federation of American Scientists, Chemical & Biological Arms Control Program [http://fas.org/bwc]
- Nat. Assoc. of County & City Health Officials [http://www.naccho.org/files/documents/responds_to_bioterrorism.html]

Academic Resources

- Johns Hopkins Center for Civilian Biodefense Studies [http://www.hopkins-biodefense.org]
- The Henry L. Stimson Center [http://www.stimson.org/cbw]
- Monterey Institute of International Studies [http://www.cns.miis.edu]
- Chemical and Biological Arms Control Institute [http://www.cbaci.org]
- UCLA Center for Public Health and Disaster Relief [http://www.ph.ucla.edu/cphdr]
- University of Minnesota Center for Infectious Disease Research and Policy [http://www1.umn.edu/cidrap]
- St. Louis University Center for the Study of Bioterrorism and Emerging Infections [http://bioterrorism.slu.edu]

Chapter 3

Bioterrorism: Summary of a CRS/National Health Policy Forum Seminar on Federal, State, and Local Public Health Preparedness[†]

Robin J. Strongin and C. Stephen Redhead

Summary

The September 11th attack and subsequent intentional release of anthrax spores via the U.S. postal system have focused policymakers' attention on the preparedness and response capability of the nation's public health system. The anthrax attacks put a tremendous strain on the U. S. public health infrastructure, an infrastructure that many experts argue has been weakened by years of neglect and under-funding. To better understand the preparedness gaps that exist, as well as the disparate functions and agencies that define public health in this country, the Congressional Research Service (CRS), in conjunction with George Washington University's National Health Policy Forum (NHPF), convened a seminar on October 26, 2001, entitled, *The U.S. Health Care System: Are State and Local Officials Prepared for Bioterrorism? How Should the Federal Government Assist?*

Speakers included William L. Roper, M.D., M.P.H., Dean, School of Public Health at the University of North Carolina; Georges C. Benjamin, M.D., Secretary, Maryland Department of Health and Mental Hygiene; Amy Smithson, Ph.D., Director, Chemical and Biological Weapons Non-Proliferation Project, the Henry L. Stimson Center; and Janet Heinrich, Dr. P.H., R.N., Director, Health Care–Public Health, U.S. General Accounting Office. The panelists presented a detailed overview of public health and the difficult choices the country faces in preparedness planning and rebuilding. The speakers made clear in their remarks that while immediate needs must be met, the importance of planning for the longer-term must not be overlooked. They suggested the need to recognize the multitude of returns on initial

---

† Excerpted from CRS Report RL31225.

investments in public health. For example, if some drug-resistant bacteria were to emerge, independent of any terrorist activity, the capabilities developed to combat bioterrorism would be invaluable.

Based upon their varied experiences, there was general consensus among all the speakers that public health preparedness, while dependent upon federal financial and other assistance, was largely a local matter. They argued that mending the gaps in the current public health fabric will require significant long-term commitments from the federal government, including investments and improvements in: laboratory capacity, regional planning, workforce training, epidemiology and surveillance systems, information systems, communication systems, and media relations.

The panelists stressed that as priorities are set and resources committed, it is imperative that all preparedness efforts be coordinated at all levels of government–federal, state, and local.

INTRODUCTION

The anthrax events that have occurred in the wake of the September 11th terrorist attacks (see box) have triggered a heightened state of alert and a series of questions related to the ability of the United States public health system to adequately meet the challenges associated with anthrax as well as smallpox, plague and other possible bioterror threat agents. In response to these questions and concerns, CRS, in conjunction with George Washington University's National Health Policy Forum, sought to provide a forum for congressional staff to hear from leading experts in the field.[1] Speakers for the session included: William L. Roper, M.D., M.P.H., Dean, School of Public Health at the University of North Carolina; Georges C. Benjamin, M.D., Secretary, Maryland Department of Health and Mental Hygiene; Amy Smithson, Ph.D., Director, Chemical and Biological Weapons Non-Proliferation Project, the Henry L. Stimson Center; and Janet Heinrich, Dr. P.H., R.N., Director, Health Care–Public Health, U.S. General Accounting Office.

Over the years, experts have been calling for a more robust public health infrastructure,[2] for a closer working relationship between the medical and public health communities, and for a broader research and development agenda in this area. Preparing for attacks that might take a number of very different forms has taken on greater urgency since September 11th. Priorities have shifted, and the importance of the public health and safety infrastructure has become a much greater concern.

---

[1] Originally conceptualized as two separate sessions, the first one focusing on the federal role in preparedness and the second on the state and local response capabilities, the meeting that ultimately took place was collapsed into one session due to the Capitol Hill closures associated with the anthrax contamination. When the meeting was finally held, it addressed both the federal as well as the state and local perspectives.

[2] The seminal 1988 Institute of Medicine (IOM) report, *The Future of Public Health* (Washington, DC: National Academy Press), identified three prongs that define public health and its infrastructure: (1) The Mission of Public Health: the fulfillment of society's interest in assuring the conditions in which people can be healthy [p. 40]; (2) The Substance of Public Health: organized community efforts aimed at the prevention of disease and promotion of health. It links many disciplines and rests upon the scientific core of epidemiology [p. 41]; and (3)The Organizational Framework of Public Health: encompasses both activities undertaken within the formal structure of government and the associated efforts of private and voluntary organizations and individuals [p. 42].

U.S. Anthrax Attacks

Twenty-two cases of anthrax have occurred as a result of the intentional dissemination of *Bacillus anthracis* spores through the U.S. postal system: 11 cases of inhalation anthrax and 11 cases (seven confirmed and four suspected) of cutaneous anthrax. Five of those with inhalation anthrax have died. The remaining 17 patients are expected to make a full recovery. The majority of cases occurred in persons working at postal facilities in New Jersey and Washington, DC, where contaminated letters were handled or processed by high-speed sorting machines, or at media companies in New York City or Florida, where the letters were delivered. At least 300 postal and other facilities have been tested for the presence of *B. anthracis* spores, and more than 32,000 potentially exposed persons have been given antibiotics.

Federal officials have confirmed that the bacterial spores used in the recent attacks in Florida, New York, and Washington, DC belong to the Ames strain, a variant of the anthrax bacterium that has been produced and studied for decades by the U.S. Army's biological weapons program. Although the Ames strain is highly virulent (i.e., effective at causing disease), it is also sensitive to a range of antibiotics. Officials have reported that the spores sent to Capitol Hill were processed into a highly concentrated and very fine, dry powder. In this form, the tiny spores, each about 1-3 microns in diameter, readily aerosolize and are capable of being inhaled deep into a person's lungs where they can trigger the most serious, inhalational-form of the disease.

Though the recent anthrax attacks are small in scale compared to the scenarios envisioned by bioterrorism experts and played out in recent government exercises (e.g., Deep Winter), they have exposed weaknesses in the public health system and shown that it is ill-prepared to deal with a large-scale bioterrorist attack.

The existence of significant gaps in the country's emergency preparedness was made clear by the speakers. Examples of the inadequacies in the public health system that emerged during the anthrax crisis included: the lack of laboratory capacity and the rapidity with which they became overwhelmed, the problems in communicating accurate information to the public, the lack of coordination and timely information exchange among the various components of the health care system, and the lack of coordination and seamless integration between public health, public safety, law enforcement, and the media. The clash of cultures – particularly around information sharing – between law enforcement (keeping information under wraps for security purposes) and public health investigations (broadly disseminating information in order to contain epidemics) was cited as having the potential to undermine the integrity and the ability of public health to accomplish its goals.

The speakers provided an overview of the current state of emergency preparedness at all levels of government, by identifying both the gaps that exist and the steps being taken to close them. A recurring theme underscored by all the presenters throughout the seminar was that closing the preparedness gaps by shoring up the public health system will help protect against the growing threat both from natural events – increasing because of global travel, ubiquitous imported food, and antibiotic resistant pathogens – as well as intentional attacks.

Key among the discussions was how to design the best preparedness "game plan." The speakers believe the plan should be: one that is well coordinated among all levels of governments and among all the various players; one that spends dollars wisely and efficiently without duplicating efforts already underway; one that depoliticizes public health and one that understands that public health is a local need dependent upon federal dollars; one that recognizes both the short and long-term needs and the fact that rural areas have even less capacity than suburban or urban areas; one that is given immediate priority.

PUBLIC HEALTH PREPAREDNESS: THIS ONE IS FOR REAL

For many years, issues pertaining to public health have seldom been given priority attention. This changed with the first case of inhalation anthrax in Florida in early October. That first case of anthrax, the index case in public health parlance, propelled the public health system into the spotlight and commanded the attention of the entire nation. Public health, explained Dr. William L. Roper,[3] is all about protecting the public against threats to their health. At the time this seminar was held, public health had become front-page news, headline information on the 24-hour news shows. But the U.S. public health infrastructure, after years of languishing was described as fragile, thin, and in need of repair. According to Dr. Roper, the nation directs most of its health resources towards medical care (e.g., physicians, hospitals) and biomedical research. The public health system receives only "crumbs," as compared to other components of the health care system.

He believes the longstanding problem of the lack of attention to and underinvestment in public health has been compounded by recent events, including pressures brought on by the current economic slowdown and state budget shortfalls. At the same time, the public health system faces increased demands and heightened expectations in the wake of September 11 and the anthrax attacks.

According to Dr. Roper, the public's expectations, not surprisingly, called for 100% protection with no risks. The goal of public health is to minimize health risks. This was a particularly challenging aspect of the anthrax events because of the unfamiliarity of the disease among medical professionals. While the science was evolving on an almost daily basis, the learning curve was steep, and public health officials and personnel – at the federal, state, and local levels – were working around the clock to try to contain the anthrax outbreaks and ease the public's fear. Dr. Roper cautioned against carping about and criticizing the Centers for Disease Control and Prevention (CDC), the lead public health agency at the federal level, and other health officials as they made their way through the nation's first major bioterror attack. While he praised the dedication of all involved, Dr. Roper voiced his concern over the inevitable emotional and physical burn-out that would ultimately occur among the front-line workers. Adding to the growing list of challenges, Dr. Roper asserted that not only would workers grow weary, but supplies of protective clothing and other gear could be depleted, further endangering health officials and first responders.

In order to meet the current public health challenges and to be better prepared for future events (which include both deliberate and naturally occurring public health threats), Dr. Roper stressed the importance of continuing the efforts already underway. Building upon existing training programs[4] (such as the Public Health Grand Rounds and the Public Health Training Network), improving existing communication systems, and strengthening existing

[3] William L. Roper, M.D., Ph.D., is Dean of the School of Public Health at the University of North Carolina. He was director of CDC from 1990–1993.

[4] For additional information, go to the University of North Carolina's School of Public Health Web site, [http://www.sph.unc.edu] and click on "bioterrorism."

information systems (such as the Health Alert Network[5]) will ultimately upgrade the public health system and infuse it with the resources, tools, and personnel that will be necessary to protect the public now and in the long-term.

PUBLIC HEALTH PREPAREDNESS: ONE STATE'S (MARYLAND) EXPERIENCE

Dr. Georges C. Benjamin[6] opened his presentation by reviewing the various types of public health concerns (organisms causing morbidity and organisms causing mortality) and the various ways in which these organisms could present, including natural events, overt events, covert events, high-risk events such as the Olympics or a presidential inaugural, and police actions that discover a risky site (e.g., finding a bioterror lab during a routine drug bust). The challenge facing public health officials is knowing when an attack has occurred, particularly in a bioterror scenario which can take days or even weeks to become obvious.

The key to preparing for such an event is surveillance – finding unprecedented numbers of cases or unusual circumstances, signs that raise the index of suspicion. The impact of surveillance on survivability is huge; Dr. Benjamin cited studies conducted by researchers at the Johns Hopkins University confirming that early warning systems save lives.

Early warning systems are one of many components necessary for successful preparedness. Disasters, Dr. Benjamin maintained, overwhelm health care systems that are already stretched thin. "One of our objectives is to shorten the time from absolute chaos to controlled disorder." Maryland has taken the following steps to better prepare for public health events, whether a naturally occurring outbreak or the result of a covert release of a dangerous pathogen.[7] These activities include:

- advance planning;
- ongoing surveillance and pre-incident intelligence gathering;
- establishing a predetermined chain of command and authority (medical personnel are not comfortable working in command and controlled environments);
- building relationships with law enforcement personnel ("have lunch with your FBI agent");
- establishing rapid, broad communication capabilities (that can identify sentinel events and enhance communications); and
- training personnel (public health staff, laboratory staff, medical providers, medical examiners, as well as mail room and office staff).

In order to minimize the chaos associated with a public health crisis, Dr. Benjamin noted that his priorities included the development of policies concerning decontamination of people

---

[5] A nationwide program, developed by the CDC in partnership with the National Association of County and City Health Officials, the Association of State and Territorial Health Officials, and other health organizations, to establish the communications, information, distance-learning, and organizational infrastructure that will link local health departments to one another and to other relevant organizations.

[6] Georges Benjamin, M.D., is Maryland's Secretary of Health and Mental Hygiene.

[7] For additional information, go to Maryland's Dept. of Health and Mental Hygiene Web site [http://www.dhmh.state.md.us].

and facilities, prophylaxis and vaccination, quarantining and isolation, and the monitoring of rescue workers. Other issues that Dr. Benjamin has planned for in order to minimize confusion during a public health crisis include: capacity building (planning for surge capacity – a sudden, often unexpected increase in service demand – among hospitals and nursing homes), preauthorization for payment (linking to managed care and other payers), community mental health needs, pest and rodent control, waste control, mortuary needs, disease follow-up, and access to vital health records.

Preparedness funding priorities for the state of Maryland center around increasing laboratory capacity (in terms of resources and personnel), strengthening communication and information systems, as well as improving training and education programs for health care workers, the public, and the media. These state set priorities mirror those articulated by Dr. Roper in his remarks. The call for better coordination, better planning, better training, as well as a greater investment in and commitment to those agencies that make up the vast network known as public health was the major theme of all four speakers.

PUBLIC HEALTH PREPAREDNESS: LESSONS FROM THE FIELD

Dr. Amy Smithson[8] drew on the research and findings from her Henry L. Stimson Center Report #35, *Ataxia: The Chemical and Biological Terrorism Threat and the U.S. Response*[9] which contained information based on the combined wisdom of front line operatives interviewed in 33 cities across the country. According to Dr. Smithson's research, most cities reported being better prepared to handle a chemical, rather than a biologic attack because cities have a sizeable number of HAZMAT (hazardous materials) teams as compared with the necessary resources that would be needed to handle a bioterror incident.

Although all those surveyed indicated an uneasiness in the level of preparedness on the "medical side of the house" for both chemical and biologic attacks, the primary concern repeatedly raised by the experts was the ability – or inability – of the cities' public health officials to be able to figure out something was wrong and to isolate the responsible organism quickly enough to be able to contain an outbreak and successfully treat the victims of such an attack.

According to experts interviewed by Dr. Smithson, disease reporting is the first critical step in determining a suspicious cluster of events. Dr. Smithson noted that the current system is reliant upon physicians who are "only human" and given the new awareness of bioterror threats, are going to be asked to identify diseases they have never seen before.

In trying to overcome this obvious hurdle, New York City (NYC) has broken new ground by monitoring all of its emergency services calls (911 calls). Analysts have developed software that can identify disease markers or sentinel events, flagging unusual outbreaks of diseases, for example during unusual seasons. If for instance, a cluster of flu-like cases were to occur during a non-peak flu season time period, this would trigger a red flag that public health officials could investigate. It is the equivalent of a digital early warning system. Over-the-counter drug products are also monitored in New York City, again to spot unusual purchasing patterns during atypical seasons. This effort requires that the resources and

[8] Amy Smithson, Ph.D., is Director of the Chemical and Biological Weapons Non-Proliferation Project at the Henry L. Stimson Center, Washington, DC.

[9] For a full copy of the report, go to [http://www.stimson.org/cwc/ataxia.htm].

capacity to harness and crunch the data are available at the local level. Similarly, New York City has also selected sentinel hospitals that are *always* on alert, always looking for the exotic disease first (an approach not typically utilized in classic diagnostic work-ups). All of these initiatives allow New York City to take the pulse of the system on a continuous basis.

Once an unusual situation is uncovered, notices can be sent out to other hospitals, laboratories, and medical personnel alerting them to a potential outbreak while at the same time seeking additional input from the field. This system is useful not just for covert criminal attacks, but is also vitally important in containing naturally occurring public health disasters such as influenza outbreaks and food-borne related illnesses. This is particularly critical given the global nature of the world today and its effect on the spread of disease.

The New York City surveillance system is unfortunately the exception and not the rule. Dr. Smithson stressed that this level of sophistication is desperately needed across the country. But, this alone is not sufficient. Dr. Smithson noted that a second tool that must be used in tandem with a sophisticated early warning surveillance system involves what a physicist at Sandia National Labs has developed. This tool is in many ways a mirror-image of the NYC system in that the capability to access data from a central data bank is placed directly in the hands of the physicians. If a patient or group of patients present with suspicious symptoms, the doctor can type data (e.g., from diagnostic tests) directly into a hand held device and retrieve information from a central data repository. Together, according to Dr. Smithson, these two tools – which would provide a rolling temporal and diagnostic map in the physician's geographic area – would arm the front line medical professionals, potentially providing enough time to jumpstart a prophylaxsis program that could save lives. The science and technology exist today to implement these capabilities. Up until very recently, however, the resources and commitment were lacking. Dr. Smithson believes that the window of opportunity to put these programs in place has never been greater.

Another largely ignored but critical component of emergency preparedness that must be improved upon is regional hospital planning. Again, according to Dr. Smithson's research, bona fide regional planning where regular disaster drills are practiced is the exception rather than the rule. During her interviews with hospital administrators, Dr. Smithson learned that the inability to charge medical personnel time to a reimbursable health service largely explained the lack of regular disaster planning and drills. Given the financial disincentives associated with these planning efforts, coupled with the relatively low level threat potential (until recently), it was not surprising that these efforts were deemed low priorities. Respondents said that most plans were drawn up using medical personnel who volunteered their time. Dr. Smithson pointed out, however, that most health professionals volunteering their time tend to work with the uninsured.

Dr. Smithson stressed that in the absence of these regional "game plans," entire local health care systems could collapse. These plans must allow for the maintenance of maternity wards, burn and trauma centers, and critical care units, services which will continue to be in demand regardless of whether a bioterror or other public health crisis ensues. Likewise, the plan must insure an adequate level of supplies (i.e., not assuming that there will be sufficient suppliers for all hospitals but actually conducting the research and mapping out the logistics of which hospital will receive what quantity of which specific supplies.) Other considerations pointed out by Dr. Smithson that warrant attention include figuring out, ahead of a crisis, precisely how the national stockpile of prescription drugs and other medical supplies will be distributed. (This aspect of planning would necessitate the provision of security in the case of mass panic.) In addition, there must be a regional plan regarding prophylaxis strategies; deciding for example, who gets vaccinated when. Another dimension requires local regions to define what assistance they can expect from the federal government, how long it will take until it arrives, and what it will take to fill the gaps until federal assistance arrives. Dr. Smithson strongly stated the opinion that while table-top exercises such as *Dark Winter* are important, they do not go nearly far enough and that it is imperative that real drills be practiced on a regular basis.[10]

Dr. Smithson made a plea to the audience that any preparedness package include adequate, well coordinated state and local public health and front line preparedness capacity building. She stressed that this does not necessarily mean more money, but money spent more wisely. She then raised the question of the role of the federal government.

PUBLIC HEALTH PREPAREDNESS: THE FEDERAL ROLE

Dr. Janet Heinrich[11] summarized the recent findings of a September 28, 2001 U.S. GAO study she directed, *Bioterrorism: Federal Research and Preparedness Activities,*[12] which found that over 20 federal agencies have a role in emergency preparedness. While the role and responsibilities of these agencies cut a wide swath, from detection of disease to the provision of vaccines, from research and development to prevention, coordination at the federal level is severely fragmented. While there are many efforts to coordinate these activities, the outlook so far, according to Dr. Heinrich, is bleak.

Pointing to the vast increase in dollars allocated to preparedness efforts (a 310% increase since FY1998) Dr. Heinrich stressed the need to establish priority spending for these monies. Her call, which was echoed by all those on the panel, was to include training, communication and information systems enhancement, and capacity building at the top of the priority list. Another important aspect of priority setting involves getting the money from the federal purse into the state and local coffers where it is needed most, in other words, deciding which priorities should be funded with federal dollars. The question was raised whether directing federal preparedness money to vaccines and prescription drug stockpiles was the most judicious use of these funds given that state and local public health entities do not rate these items high on their priority lists. GAO found that vaccine and drug stockpiles are seen by many public health officials in the trenches as a short-term "band-aid" fix for a limited number of biologic threats, and not the crucial longer-term commitment needed to shore up the thinly stretched basic public health infrastructure of today. It was pointed out that one key contribution the new office of homeland security could make would be to assist in coordinating the transfer of federal dollars to local level needs.

[10] Dark Winter was an exercise designed to simulate possible U.S. reaction to the deliberate introduction of smallpox in 3 states during the winter of 2002. The exercise itself was conducted at Andrews Air Force Base on June 22–23, 2001. Former senior government officials played the roles of National Security Council members responding to the evolving epidemic. For more information on Dark Winter, go to [http://www.hopkins-biodefense.org].

[11] Janet Heinrich, Dr.P.H., R.N., is Director of Health Care and Public Health issues at the U.S. General Accounting Office.

[12] A copy of the report in its entirety can be found by going to the GAO Web site [http://www.gao.gov], clicking on "Find GAO Reports" and entering report number "GAO-01-915."

QUESTIONS FROM THE AUDIENCE

Questions from the audience covered several themes, most of which revolved around the division of labor and responsibility among the federal, state, and local governments. One audience member questioned whether today's decentralized public health system is the most appropriate structure for fighting the war on terrorism. It was pointed out that the recent terror attacks were really national attacks, akin in many ways to the attack on Pearl Harbor (in which a national response ensued). The consensus among the panelists was that these issues are local and that a national superstructure would ultimately create a false sense of security and would undermine the ability of an already fractured local public health system to rebuild. The panelists were of the strong opinion that this is *the* opportunity for shoring up and bolstering a permanent state and local capacity and that there was a definite role for the federal government, one that was not solely centered on finances. An example cited was that while the CDC is only one component of the U.S. public health enterprise, it is a vital resource to state and local officials. If, however, experts at the CDC are prohibited from sharing information, the integrity and the ability of the entire public health infrastructure could be at stake. So too might be the health of the public.

Another area that received attention from the audience involved states' capacities to effectively use additional funds that would make their way from the federal coffers into state and local budgets. Concern was expressed among many in the audience that there be adequate accountability as to how the new federal dollars would be spent in the name of bioterror and emergency preparedness. Monies should not be diverted to oncology wards, for example, at the expense of decontamination units.

The issue of incorporating professional standards for front line and medical personnel into education programs was raised in a related round of questions and answers. The panel agreed that where the power of Washington could be brought to bear was in institutionalizing professional standards into existing programs that could be modified to incorporate bioterrorism training. They said it would not be enough for the federal government to dictate exactly how to conduct a particular preparedness related activity. Rather, the states should be given maximum flexibility and control, but at the same time, they must be held accountable.

There seemed to be agreement that while most of the day to day action would continue to take place at the state and local levels, there were several important ways the federal government could enhance preparedness (e.g., financing and conducting technical research and development, financing and maintaining the national pharmaceutical stockpile and coordinating and sharing clinical expertise through the CDC). But to be successful, such commitment must not waver when the anthrax crisis comes to a close. An example of "yo-yo public health funding" commitments cited was the U.S. experience with tuberculosis (TB). When the country faced a serious TB epidemic, monies were provided with the express purpose of ridding the country of TB. But as soon as TB was largely eradicated, the monies were cut. The lack of public health funds for education and prevention contributed to the return of TB, only this time it came back in an antibiotic-resistant form. More monies had to be infused into the system, and eradicating antibiotic-resistant TB remains a public health challenge. The message from the speakers was clear: fighting disease – whether naturally occurring or manmade – will require a consistent, coordinated, long-term commitment.

CONCLUSION

The distinction between bioterrorism and chemical terrorism, as well as that between radiologic and nuclear terrorism, is critical, for in the differences between them lie the unique requirements for preparedness. While many of the issues and challenges are the same, regardless of the type of terror attack (for example, the ability of the health care system to deal with mass casualties and the "worried well," short and long-term mental health needs, and panic), the nature of an attack will determine the needed response and ultimately the level of preparedness. In the end, while the initial responses may start out differently, all emergency responses ultimately rely on the same health and safety infrastructure. An infrastructure which has fallen into a critical state of disrepair after years of neglect and budget cuts, according to the speakers at the seminar. As federal and state lawmakers debate and devise strategies for becoming better prepared, there was consensus among all the panelists that whatever form the final plans take, they should be well coordinated, well funded, and long-term.

Chapter 4

BIOTERRORISM: PUBLIC HEALTH AND MEDICAL PREPAREDNESS[‡]

Janet Heinrich

In this chapter discussed is the GAO's work on the activities of federal agencies to prepare the nation to respond to the public health and medical consequences of a bioterrorist attack.[1] Preparing to respond to the public health and medical consequences of a bioterrorist attack poses some challenges that are different from those in other types of terrorist attacks, such as bombings. On September 28, 2001, we released a report[2] that describes (1) the research and preparedness activities being undertaken by federal departments and agencies to manage the consequences of a bioterrorist attack,[3] (2) the coordination of these activities, and (3) the findings of reports on the preparedness of state and local jurisdictions to respond to a bioterrorist attack. Summarized are the detailed findings included in our report, highlighting weaknesses in the public health infrastructure that we have identified in our ongoing work and which we believe warrant special attention.

In summary, we identified more than 20 federal departments and agencies as having a role in preparing for or responding to the public health and medical consequences of a bioterrorist attack. These agencies are participating in a variety of activities, from improving the detection of biological agents to developing a national stockpile of pharmaceuticals to treat victims of disasters. Federal departments and agencies have engaged in a number of

---

‡ *Testimony before the Subcommittee on Public Health, Committee on Health, Education, Labor, and Pensions, United States Senate. October 9, 2001.* Excerpted from GAO Report GAO-02-141T.

1 Bioterrorism is the threat or intentional release of biological agents (viruses, bacteria, or their toxins) for the purposes of influencing the conduct of government or intimidating or coercing a civilian population.

2 See Bioterrorism: Federal Research and Preparedness Activities (GAO-01-915, Sept. 28, 2001). This report was mandated by the Public Health Improvement Act of 2000 (P.L. 106-505, sec. 102). Also, see the list of related GAO products at the end of this statement.

3 We conducted interviews with and obtained information from the Departments of Agriculture, Commerce, Defense, Energy, Health and Human Services, Justice, Transportation, the Treasury, and Veterans Affairs; the Environmental Protection Agency; and the Federal Emergency Management Agency.

efforts to coordinate these activities on a formal and informal basis, such as interagency work groups. Despite these efforts, we found evidence that coordination between departments and agencies is fragmented. We did, however, find recent actions to improve coordination across federal departments and agencies. In addition, we found emerging concerns about the preparedness of state and local jurisdictions, including insufficient state and local planning for response to terrorist events, a lack of hospital participation in training on terrorism and emergency response planning, the timely availability of medical teams and resources in an emergency, and inadequacies in the public health infrastructure. The last includes weaknesses in the training of health care providers, communication among responsible parties, and capacity of laboratories and hospitals, including the ability to treat mass casualties.

BACKGROUND

A domestic bioterrorist attack is considered to be a low-probability event, in part because of the various difficulties involved in successfully delivering biological agents to achieve large-scale casualties.[4] However, a number of cases involving biological agents, including at least one completed bioterrorist act and numerous threats and hoaxes,[5] have occurred domestically. In 1984, a group intentionally contaminated salad bars in restaurants in Oregon with salmonella bacteria. Although no one died, 751 people were diagnosed with foodborne illness. Some experts predict that more domestic bioterrorist attacks are likely to occur.

The burden of responding to such an attack would fall initially on personnel in state and local emergency response agencies. These "first responders" include firefighters, emergency medical service personnel, law enforcement officers, public health officials, health care workers (including doctors, nurses, and other medical professionals), and public works personnel. If the emergency were to require federal disaster assistance, federal departments and agencies would respond according to responsibilities outlined in the Federal Response Plan.[6] Several groups, including the Advisory Panel to Assess Domestic Response Capabilities for Terrorism Involving Weapons of Mass Destruction (known as the Gilmore Panel), have assessed the capabilities at the federal, state, and local levels to respond to a domestic terrorist incident involving a weapon of mass destruction (WMD), that is, a chemical, biological, radiological, or nuclear agent or weapon.[7]

While many aspects of an effective response to bioterrorism are the same as those for any disaster, there are some unique features. For example, if a biological agent is released covertly, it may not be recognized for a week or more because symptoms may not appear for

[4] See Combating Terrorism: Need for Comprehensive Threat and Risk Assessments of Chemical and Biological Attacks (GAO/NSIAD-99-163, Sept. 14, 1999), pp. 10-15, for a discussion of the ease or difficulty for a terrorist to create mass casualties by making or using chemical or biological agents without the assistance of a state-sponsored program.

[5] For example, in January 2000, threatening letters were sent to a variety of recipients, including the Planned Parenthood office in Naples, Florida, warning of the release of anthrax. Federal authorities found no signs of anthrax or any other traces of harmful substances and determined these incidences to be hoaxes.

[6] The Federal Response Plan, originally drafted in 1992 and updated in 1999, is authorized under the Robert T. Stafford Disaster Relief and Emergency Assistance Act (Stafford Act; P.L. 93-288, as amended). The plan outlines the planning assumptions, policies, concept of operations, organizational structures, and specific assignment of responsibilities to lead departments and agencies in providing federal assistance once the President has declared an emergency requiring federal assistance.

[7] Some agencies define WMDs to include large conventional explosives as well.

several days after the initial exposure and may be misdiagnosed at first. In addition, some biological agents, such as smallpox, are communicable and can spread to others who were not initially exposed. These differences require a type of response that is unique to bioterrorism, including infectious disease surveillance,[8] epidemiologic investigation,[9] laboratory identification of biological agents, and distribution of antibiotics to large segments of the population to prevent the spread of an infectious disease. However, some aspects of an effective response to bioterrorism are also important in responding to any type of large-scale disaster, such as providing emergency medical services, continuing health care services delivery, and managing mass fatalities.

FEDERAL DEPARTMENTS AND AGENCIES REPORTED A VARIETY OF RESEARCH AND PREPAREDNESS ACTIVITIES

Federal spending on domestic preparedness for terrorist attacks involving WMDs has risen 310 percent since fiscal year 1998, to approximately $1.7 billion in fiscal year 2001, and may increase significantly after the events of September 11, 2001. However, only a portion of these funds were used to conduct a variety of activities related to research on and preparedness for the public health and medical consequences of a bioterrorist attack. We cannot measure the total investment in such activities because departments and agencies provided funding information in various forms—as appropriations, obligations, or expenditures. Because the funding information provided is not equivalent,[10] we summarized funding by department or agency, but not across the federal government (see apps. I and II).[11] Reported funding generally shows increases from fiscal year 1998 to fiscal year 2001. Several agencies received little or no funding in fiscal year 1998. For example, within the Department of Health and Human Services (HHS), the Centers for Disease Control and Prevention's (CDC) Bioterrorism Preparedness and Response Program was established and first received funding in fiscal year 1999 (see app. I and app. II). Its funding has increased from approximately $121 million at that time to approximately $194 million in fiscal year 2001.

---

[8] Disease surveillance systems provide for the ongoing collection, analysis, and dissemination of data to prevent and control disease.

[9] Epidemiological investigation is the study of patterns of health or disease and the factors that influence these patterns.

[10] For example, an agency providing appropriations is not necessarily indicating the level of its commitments (that is, obligations) or expenditures for that year—only the amount of budget authority made available to it by the Congress, some of which may be unspent. Similarly, an agency that provided expenditure information for fiscal year 2000 may have obligated the funds in fiscal year 1999 based on an appropriation for fiscal year 1998. To simplify presentation, we generally refer to all the budget data we received from agencies as "reported funding."

[11] Although there are generally no specific appropriations for activities on bioterrorism, some departments and agencies did provide estimates of the funds they were devoting to activities on bioterrorism. Other departments and agencies provided estimates for overall terrorism activities, but were unable to provide funding amounts for activities on bioterrorism specifically. Still others stated that their activities were relevant for bioterrorism, but they were unable to specify the funding amounts. Funding levels for activities on terrorism, including bioterrorism, were reported for activities prior to the 2001 Emergency Supplemental Appropriations Act for Recovery From and Response to Terrorist Attacks on the United States (P.L. 107-38).

Research Activities Focus on Detection, Treatment, Vaccination and Equipment

Research is currently being done to enable the rapid identification of biological agents in a variety of settings; develop new or improved vaccines, antibiotics, and antivirals to improve treatment and vaccination for infectious diseases caused by biological agents; and develop and test emergency response equipment such as respiratory and other personal protective equipment. Appendix I provides information on the total reported funding for all the departments and agencies carrying out research, along with examples of this research.

The Department of Agriculture (USDA), Department of Defense (DOD), Department of Energy, HHS, Department of Justice (DOJ), Department of the Treasury, and the Environmental Protection Agency (EPA) have all sponsored or conducted projects to improve the detection and characterization of biological agents in a variety of different settings, from water to clinical samples (such as blood). For example, EPA is sponsoring research to improve its ability to detect biological agents in the water supply. Some of these projects, such as those conducted or sponsored by DOD and DOJ, are not primarily for the public health and medical consequences of a bioterrorist attack against the civilian population, but could eventually benefit research for those purposes.

Departments and agencies are also conducting or sponsoring studies to improve treatment and vaccination for diseases caused by biological agents. For example, HHS' projects include basic research sponsored by the National Institutes of Health to develop drugs and diagnostics and applied research sponsored by the Agency for Healthcare Research and Quality to improve health care delivery systems by studying the use of information systems and decision support systems to enhance preparedness for the delivery of medical care in an emergency.

In addition, several agencies, including the Department of Commerce's National Institute of Standards and Technology and DOJ's National Institute of Justice are conducting research that focuses on developing performance standards and methods for testing the performance of emergency response equipment, such as respirators and personal protective equipment.

Preparedness Efforts Include Multiple Actions

Federal departments' and agencies' preparedness efforts have included efforts to increase federal, state, and local response capabilities, develop response teams of medical professionals, increase availability of medical treatments, participate in and sponsor terrorism response exercises, plan to aid victims, and provide support during special events such as presidential inaugurations, major political party conventions, and the Superbowl.[12] Appendix II contains information on total reported funding for all the departments and agencies with bioterrorism preparedness activities, along with examples of these activities.

Several federal departments and agencies, such as the Federal Emergency Management Agency (FEMA) and CDC, have programs to increase the ability of state and local authorities to successfully respond to an emergency, including a bioterrorist attack. These departments and agencies contribute to state and local jurisdictions by helping them pay for equipment and

[12] Presidential Decision Directive 62, issued May 22, 1998, created a category of special events called National Security Special Events, which are events of such significance that they warrant greater federal planning and protection than other special events.

develop emergency response plans, providing technical assistance, increasing communications capabilities, and conducting training courses.

Federal departments and agencies have also been increasing their own capacity to identify and deal with a bioterrorist incident. For example, CDC, USDA, and the Food and Drug Administration (FDA) are improving surveillance methods for detecting disease outbreaks in humans and animals. They have also established laboratory response networks to maintain state-of-the-art capabilities for biological agent identification and the characterization of human clinical samples.

Some federal departments and agencies have developed teams to directly respond to terrorist events and other emergencies. For example, HHS' Office of Emergency Preparedness (OEP) created Disaster Medical Assistance Teams to provide medical treatment and assistance in the event of an emergency. Four of these teams, known as National Medical Response Teams, are specially trained and equipped to provide medical care to victims of WMD events, such as bioterrorist attacks.

Several agencies are involved in increasing the availability of medical supplies that could be used in an emergency, including a bioterrorist attack. CDC's National Pharmaceutical Stockpile contains pharmaceuticals, antidotes, and medical supplies that can be delivered anywhere in the United States within 12 hours of the decision to deploy. The stockpile was deployed for the first time on September 11, 2001, in response to the terrorist attacks on New York City.

Federally initiated bioterrorism response exercises have been conducted across the country. For example, in May 2000, many departments and agencies took part in the Top Officials 2000 exercise (TOPOFF 2000) in Denver, Colorado, which featured the simulated release of a biological agent.[13] Participants included local fire departments, police, hospitals, the Colorado Department of Public Health and the Environment, the Colorado Office of Emergency Management, the Colorado National Guard, the American Red Cross, the Salvation Army, HHS, DOD, FEMA, the Federal Bureau of Investigation (FBI), and EPA.

Several agencies also provide assistance to victims of terrorism. FEMA can provide supplemental funds to state and local mental health agencies for crisis counseling to eligible survivors of presidentially declared emergencies. In the aftermath of the recent terrorist attacks, HHS released $1 million in funding to New York State to support mental health services and strategic planning for comprehensive and long-term support to address the mental health needs of the community. DOJ's Office of Justice Programs (OJP) also manages a program that provides funds for victims of terrorist attacks that can be used to provide a variety of services, including mental health treatment and financial assistance to attend related criminal proceedings.

Federal departments and agencies also provide support at special events to improve response in case of an emergency. For example, CDC has deployed a system to provide increased surveillance and epidemiological capacity before, during, and after special events. Besides improving emergency response at the events, participation by departments and agencies gives them valuable experience working together to develop and practice plans to combat terrorism.

---

[13] In addition to simulating a bioterrorism attack in Denver, the exercise also simulated a chemical weapons incident in Portsmouth, New Hampshire. A concurrent exercise, referred to as National Capital Region 2000, simulated a radiological event in the greater Washington, D.C., area.

FRAGMENTATION REMAINS DESPITE EFFORTS TO COORDINATE FEDERAL PROGRAMS

Federal departments and agencies are using a variety of interagency plans, work groups, and agreements to coordinate their activities to combat terrorism. However, we found evidence that coordination remains fragmented. For example, several different agencies are responsible for various coordination functions, which limits accountability and hinders unity of effort; several key agencies have not been included in bioterrorism-related policy and response planning; and the programs that agencies have developed to provide assistance to state and local governments are similar and potentially duplicative. The President recently took steps to improve oversight and coordination, including the creation of the Office of Homeland Security.

Departments and Agencies Use a Variety of Methods to Coordinate Activities

Over 40 federal departments and agencies have some role in combating terrorism, and coordinating their activities is a significant challenge. We identified over 20 departments and agencies as having a role in preparing for or responding to the public health and medical consequences of a bioterrorist attack. Appendix III, which is based on the framework given in the Terrorism Incident Annex of the Federal Response Plan, shows a sample of the coordination efforts by federal departments and agencies with responsibilities for the public health and medical consequences of a bioterrorist attack, as they existed prior to the recent creation of the Office of Homeland Security. This figure illustrates the complex relationships among the many federal departments and agencies involved.

Departments and agencies use several approaches to coordinate their activities on terrorism, including interagency response plans, work groups, and formal agreements. Interagency plans for responding to a terrorist incident help outline agency responsibilities and identify resources that could be used during a response. For example, the Federal Response Plan provides a broad framework for coordinating the delivery of federal disaster assistance to state and local governments when an emergency overwhelms their ability to respond effectively. The Federal Response Plan also designates primary and supporting federal agencies for a variety of emergency support operations. For example, HHS is the primary agency for coordinating federal assistance in response to public health and medical care needs in an emergency. HHS could receive support from other agencies and organizations, such as DOD, USDA, and FEMA, to assist state and local jurisdictions.

Interagency work groups are being used to minimize duplication of funding and effort in federal activities to combat terrorism. For example, the Technical Support Working Group is chartered to coordinate interagency research and development requirements across the federal government in order to prevent duplication of effort between agencies. The Technical Support Working Group, among other projects, helped to identify research needs and fund a project to detect biological agents in food that can be used by both DOD and USDA.

Formal agreements between departments and agencies are being used to share resources and knowledge. For example, CDC contracts with the Department of Veterans Affairs (VA) to purchase drugs and medical supplies for the National Pharmaceutical Stockpile because of VA's purchasing power and ability to negotiate large discounts.

Coordination Remains Fragmented Within the Federal Government

Overall coordination of federal programs to combat terrorism is fragmented.[14] For example, several agencies have coordination functions, including DOJ, the FBI, FEMA, and the Office of Management and Budget. Officials from a number of the agencies that combat terrorism told us that the coordination roles of these various agencies are not always clear and sometimes overlap, leading to a fragmented approach. We have found that the overall coordination of federal research and development efforts to combat terrorism is still limited by several factors, including the compartmentalization or security classification of some research efforts.[15] The Gilmore Panel also concluded that the current coordination structure does not provide for the requisite authority or accountability to impose the discipline necessary among the federal agencies involved.[16]

The multiplicity of federal assistance programs requires focus and attention to minimize redundancy of effort.[17] Table 1 shows some of the federal programs providing assistance to state and local governments for emergency planning that would be relevant to responding to a bioterrorist attack. While the programs vary somewhat in their target audiences, the potential redundancy of these federal efforts highlights the need for scrutiny. In our report on combating terrorism, issued on September 20, 2001, we recommended that the President, working closely with the Congress, consolidate some of the activities of DOJ's OJP under FEMA.[18]

[14] See also Combating Terrorism: Comments on Counterterrorism Leadership and National Strategy (GAO-01-556T, Mar. 27, 2001), p. 1.

[15] See Combating Terrorism: Selected Challenges and Related Recommendations (GAO-01-822, Sept. 20, 2001), pp. 79, 84.

[16] Advisory Panel to Assess Domestic Response Capabilities for Terrorism Involving Weapons of Mass Destruction (Gilmore Panel), Toward a National Strategy for Combating Terrorism, Second Annual Report (Arlington, Va.: RAND, Dec. 15, 2000), p. 7.

[17] See also Combating Terrorism: Issues in Managing Counterterrorist Programs (GAO/T-NSIAD-00-145, Apr. 6, 2000), p. 8.

[18] See GAO-01-822, Sept. 20, 2001, pp. 104-106.

Table 1: Selected Federal Activities Providing Assistance to State and Local Governments for Emergency Planning Relevant to a Bioterrorist Attack

Department or agency	Activities	Target audience
HHS—CDC	Provides grants, technical support, and performance standards to support bioterrorism preparedness and response planning.	State and local health agencies
HHS—OEP	Enters into contracts to enhance medical response capability. The program includes a focus on response to bioterrorism, including early recognition, mass postexposure treatment, mass casualty care, and mass fatality management.	Local jurisdictions (for fire, police, and emergency medical services; hospitals; public health agencies; and other services)
DOJ—OJP	Assists states in developing strategic plans. Includes funding for training, equipment acquisition, technical assistance, and exercise planning and execution to enhance state and local capabilities to respond to terrorist incidents.	States (for fire, law enforcement, emergency medical, and hazardous materials response services; hospitals; public health departments; and other services)
FEMA	Provides grant assistance to support state and local consequence management planning, training, and exercises for all types of terrorism, including bioterrorism.	State emergency management agencies

Source: Information obtained from departments and agencies.

We have also recommended that the federal government conduct multidisciplinary and analytically sound threat and risk assessments to define and prioritize requirements and properly focus programs and investments in combating terrorism.[19] Such assessments would be useful in addressing the fragmentation that is evident in the different threat lists of biological agents developed by federal departments and agencies.

Understanding which biological agents are considered most likely to be used in an act of domestic terrorism is necessary to focus the investment in new technologies, equipment, training, and planning. Several different agencies have or are in the process of developing biological agent threat lists, which differ based on the agencies' focus. For example, CDC collaborated with law enforcement, intelligence, and defense agencies to develop a critical agent list that focuses on the biological agents that would have the greatest impact on public health. The FBI, the National Institute of Justice, and the Technical Support Working Group are completing a report that lists biological agents that may be more likely to be used by a terrorist group working in the United States that is not sponsored by a foreign government. In addition, an official at USDA's Animal and Plant Health Inspection Service told us that it uses two lists of agents of concern for a potential bioterrorist attack. These lists of agents, only some of which are capable of making both animals and humans sick, were developed

[19] See Combating Terrorism: Threat and Risk Assessments Can Help Prioritize and Target Program Investments (GAO/NSIAD-98-74, Apr. 9, 1998) and GAO/NSIAD-99-163, Sept. 14, 1999.

through an international process. According to agency officials, separate threat lists are appropriate because of the different focuses of these agencies. In our view, the existence of competing lists makes the assignment of priorities difficult for state and local officials.

Fragmentation is also apparent in the composition of groups of federal agencies involved in bioterrorism-related planning and policy. Officials at the Department of Transportation (DOT) told us that that even though the nation's transportation centers account for a significant percentage of the nation's potential terrorist targets, the department was not part of the founding group of agencies that worked on bioterrorism issues and has not been included in bioterrorism response plans. DOT officials also told us that the department is supposed to deliver supplies for FEMA under the Federal Response Plan, but it was not brought into the planning early enough to understand the extent of its responsibilities in the transportation process. The department learned what its responsibilities would be during the TOPOFF 2000 exercise, which simulated a release of a biological agent.

Recent Actions Seek to Improve Coordination Across Federal Departments and Agencies

In May 2001, the President asked the Vice President to oversee the development of a coordinated national effort dealing with WMDs.[20] At the same time, the President asked the Director of FEMA to establish an Office of National Preparedness to implement the results of the Vice President's effort that relate to programs within federal agencies that address consequence management resulting from the use of WMDs. The purpose of this effort is to better focus policies and ensure that programs and activities are fully coordinated in support of building the needed preparedness and response capabilities. In addition, on September 20, 2001, the President announced the creation of the Office of Homeland Security to lead, oversee, and coordinate a comprehensive national strategy to protect the country from terrorism and respond to any attacks that may occur. These actions represent potentially significant steps toward improved coordination of federal activities. Our recent report highlighted a number of important characteristics and responsibilities necessary for a single focal point, such as the proposed Office of Homeland Security, to improve coordination and accountability.[21]

Despite Federal Efforts, Concerns Exist Regarding Preparedness at State and Local Levels

Nonprofit research organizations, congressionally chartered advisory panels, government documents, and articles in peer-reviewed literature have identified concerns about the preparedness of states and local areas to respond to a bioterrorist attack. These concerns include insufficient state and local planning for response to terrorist events, a lack of hospital participation in training on terrorism and emergency response planning, questions regarding

---

[20] According to the Office of the Vice President, as of June 2001, details on the Vice President's efforts had not yet been determined.

[21] See GAO-01-822, Sept. 20, 2001, pp. 41-42.

the timely availability of medical teams and resources in an emergency, and inadequacies in the public health infrastructure. In our view, there are weaknesses in three key areas of the public health infrastructure: training of health care providers, communication among responsible parties, and capacity of laboratories and hospitals, including the ability to treat mass casualties.

Questions exist regarding how effectively federal programs have prepared state and local governments to respond to terrorism. All 50 states and approximately 255 local jurisdictions have received or are scheduled to receive at least some federal assistance, including training and equipment grants, to help them prepare for a terrorist WMD incident. In 1997, FEMA identified planning and equipment for response to nuclear, biological, and chemical incidents as areas in need of significant improvement at the state level. However, an October 2000 research report concluded that even those cities receiving federal aid are still not adequately prepared to respond to a bioterrorist attack.[22]

Inadequate training and planning for bioterrorism response by hospitals is a major problem. The Gilmore Panel concluded that the level of expertise in recognizing and dealing with a terrorist attack involving a biological or chemical agent is problematic in many hospitals.[23] A recent research report concluded that hospitals need to improve their preparedness for mass casualty incidents.[24] Local officials told us that it has been difficult to get hospitals and medical personnel to participate in local training, planning, and exercises to improve their preparedness.

Local officials are also concerned about whether the federal government could quickly deliver enough medical teams and resources to help after a biological attack.[25] Agency officials say that federal response teams, such as Disaster Medical Assistance Teams, could be on site within 12 to 24 hours. However, local officials who have deployed with such teams say that the federal assistance probably would not arrive for 24 to 72 hours. Local officials also told us that they were concerned about the time and resources required to prepare and distribute drugs from the National Pharmaceutical Stockpile during an emergency. Partially in response to these concerns, CDC has developed training for state and local officials in using the stockpile and will deploy a small staff with the supplies to assist the local jurisdiction with distribution.

Components of the nation's public health system are also not well prepared to detect or respond to a bioterrorist attack. In particular, weaknesses exist in the key areas of training, communication, and hospital and laboratory capacity. It has been reported that physicians and nurses in emergency rooms and private offices, who will most likely be the first health care workers to see patients following a bioterrorist attack, lack the needed training to ensure their ability to make observations of unusual symptoms and patterns.[26] Most physicians and nurses have never seen cases of certain diseases, such as smallpox or plague, and some biological agents initially produce symptoms that can be easily confused with influenza or other, less virulent illnesses, leading to a delay in diagnosis or identification. Medical laboratory

[22] A.E. Smithson and L.-A. Levy, Ataxia: The Chemical and Biological Terrorism Threat and the U.S. Response (Washington, D.C.: The Henry L. Stimson Center, Oct. 2000), p. 271.

[23] Advisory Panel to Assess Domestic Response Capabilities for Terrorism Involving Weapons of Mass Destruction, p. 32.

[24] D.C. Wetter, W.E. Daniell, and C.D. Treser, "Hospital Preparedness for Victims of Chemical or Biological Terrorism," American Journal of Public Health, Vol. 91, No. 5 (May 2001), pp. 710-16.

[25] Smithson and Levy, p. 227.

[26] Smithson and Levy, p. 248.

personnel require training because they also lack experience in identifying biological agents such as anthrax.

Because it could take days to weeks to identify the pathogen used in a biological attack, good channels of communication among the parties involved in the response are essential to ensure that the response proceeds as rapidly as possible. Physicians will need to report their observations to the infectious disease surveillance system. Once the disease outbreak has been recognized, local health departments will need to collaborate closely with personnel across a variety of agencies to bring in the needed expertise and resources. They will need to obtain the information necessary to conduct epidemiological investigations to establish the likely site and time of exposure, the size and location of the exposed population, and the prospects for secondary transmission. However, past experiences with infectious disease response have revealed a lack of sufficient and secure channels for sharing information. Our report last year on the initial West Nile virus outbreak in New York City found that as the public health investigation grew, lines of communication were often unclear, and efforts to keep everyone informed were awkward, such as conference calls that lasted for hours and involved dozens of people.[27]

Adequate laboratory and hospital capacity is also a concern. Reductions in public health laboratory staffing and training have affected the ability of state and local authorities to identify biological agents. Even the initial West Nile virus outbreak in 1999, which was relatively small and occurred in an area with one of the nation's largest local public health agencies, taxed the federal, state, and local laboratory resources. Both the New York State and the CDC laboratories were inundated with requests for tests, and the CDC laboratory handled the bulk of the testing because of the limited capacity at the New York laboratories. Officials indicated that the CDC laboratory would have been unable to respond to another outbreak, had one occurred at the same time. In fiscal year 2000, CDC awarded approximately $11 million to 48 states and four major urban health departments to improve and upgrade their surveillance and epidemiological capabilities. With regard to hospitals, several federal and local officials reported that there is little excess capacity in the health care system in most communities for accepting and treating mass casualty patients. Research reports have concluded that the patient load of a regular influenza season in the late 1990s overtaxed primary care facilities and that emergency rooms in major metropolitan areas are routinely filled and unable to accept patients in need of urgent care.[28]

Concluding Observations

We found that federal departments and agencies are participating in a variety of research and preparedness activities that are important steps in improving our readiness. Although federal departments and agencies have engaged in a number of efforts to coordinate these activities on a formal and informal basis, we found that coordination between departments

---

[27] See West Nile Virus Outbreak: Lessons for Public Health Preparedness (GAO/HEHS-00-180, Sept. 11, 2000), pp. 21-22.

[28] J.R. Richards, M.L. Navarro, and R.W. Derlet, "Survey of Directors of Emergency Departments in California on Overcrowding," Western Journal of Medicine, Vol. 172 (June 2000), pp. 385-88. R. Derlet, J. Richards, and R. Kravitz, "Frequent Overcrowding in U.S. Emergency Departments," Academic Emergency Medicine, Vol. 8, No. 2 (2001), pp.151-55. Smithson and Levy, p. 262.

and agencies is fragmented. In addition, we remain concerned about weaknesses in public health preparedness at the state and local levels, a lack of hospital participation in training on terrorism and emergency response planning, the timely availability of medical teams and resources in an emergency, and, in particular, inadequacies in the public health infrastructure. The latter include weaknesses in the training of health care providers, communication among responsible parties, and capacity of laboratories and hospitals, including the ability to treat mass casualties.

APPENDIX I: FUNDING FOR RESEARCH

Total Reported Funding for Research on Bioterrorism and Terrorism by Federal Departments and Agencies, Fiscal Year 2000 and Fiscal Year 2001

Dollars in millions

Department or agency	Fiscal year 2000 funding	Fiscal year 2001 funding	Sample activities
U.S. Department of Agriculture (USDA)—Agricultural Research Service	0	$0.5	Improving detection of biological agents
Department of Energy	$35.5	$39.6	Developing technologies for detecting and responding to a bioterrorist attack Developing models of the spread of and exposure to a biological agent after release
Department of Health and Human Services (HHS)—Agency for Healthcare Research and Quality	$5.0	0	Examining clinical training and ability of frontline medical staff to detect and respond to a bioterrorist threat Studying use of information systems and decision support systems to enhance preparedness for medical care in the event of a bioterrorist event
HHS—Centers for Disease Control and Prevention (CDC)	$48.2	$46.6	Developing equipment performance standards Conducting research on smallpox and anthrax viruses and therapeutics
HHS—Food and Drug Administration (FDA)	$8.8	$9.1	Licensing of vaccines for anthrax and smallpox Determining procedures for allowing use of not-yet-approved drugs and specifying data needed for approval and labeling
HHS—National Institutes of Health	$43.0	$49.7	Developing new therapies for smallpox virus Developing smallpox and bacterial antigen detection system
HHS—Office of Emergency Preparedness (OEP)	0	$4.6	Overseeing a study on response systems
Department of Justice (DOJ)—Office of Justice Programs (OJP)	$0.7	$4.6	Developing a biological agent detector
DOJ—Federal Bureau of Investigation	0	$1.1	Conducting work on detection and characterization of biological materials
Department of the Treasury—Secret Service	0	$0.5	Developing a biological agent detector
Environmental Protection Agency (EPA)	0	$0.5	Improving detection of biological agents

Note: Total reported funding refers to budget data we received from agencies. Agencies reported appropriations, actual or estimated obligations, or actual or estimated expenditures. An agency providing appropriations is not necessarily indicating the level of its obligations or expenditures for that year—only the amount of budget authority made available to it by the Congress. Similarly, an agency that provided expenditure information for fiscal year 2000 may have obligated the funds in fiscal year 1999 based on an appropriation for fiscal year 1998.

Source: Information obtained from departments and agencies.

APPENDIX II: FUNDING FOR PREPAREDNESS ACTIVITIES

Total Reported Funding for Preparedness Activities on Bioterrorism and Terrorism by Federal Departments and Agencies, Fiscal Year 2000 and Fiscal Year 2001

Dollars in millions

Department or agency	Fiscal year 2000 funding	Fiscal year 2001 funding	Sample activities
USDA—Animal and Plant Health Inspection Service	0	$0.2	Developing educational materials and training programs specifically dealing with bioterrorism
Department of Defense (DOD)—Joint Task Force for Civil Support	$3.4	$8.7	Planning, and when directed, commanding and controlling DOD's WMD and high-yield explosive consequence management capabilities in support of FEMA
DOD—National Guard	$70.0	$93.3	Managing response teams that would enter a contaminated area to gather samples for on-site evaluation
DOD—U.S. Army	$29.5	$11.7	Maintaining a repository of information about chemical and biological weapons and agents, detectors, and protection and decontamination equipment
HHS—CDC	$124.9	$147.3	Awarding planning grants to state and local health departments to prepare bioterrorism response plans Improving surveillance methods for detecting disease outbreaks Increasing communication capabilities in order to improve the gathering and exchanging of information related to bioterrorist incidents
HHS—FDA	$0.1	$2.1	Improving capabilities to identify and characterize foodborne pathogens Identifying biological agents using animal studies and microbiological surveillance
HHS—OEP	$35.3	$46.1	Providing contracts to increase local emergency response capabilities Developing and managing response teams that can provide support at the site of a disaster
DOJ—OJP	$7.6	$5.3	Helping prepare state and local emergency responders through training, exercises, technical assistance, and equipment programs Developing a data collection tool to assist states in conducting their threat, risk, and needs assessments, and in developing their preparedness strategy for terrorism, including bioterrorism
EPA	$0.1	$2.0	Providing technical assistance in identifying biological agents and decontaminating affected areas Conducting assessments of water supply vulnerability to terrorism, including contamination with biological agents
Federal Emergency Management Agency	$25.1	$30.3	Providing grant assistance and guidance to states for planning and training Maintaining databases of safety precautions for biological, chemical, and nuclear agents

Note: Total reported funding refers to budget data we received from agencies. Agencies reported appropriations, actual or estimated obligations, or actual or estimated expenditures. An agency providing appropriations is not necessarily indicating the level of its obligations or expenditures for that year—only the amount of budget authority made available to it by the Congress. Similarly, an agency that provided expenditure information for fiscal year 2000 may have obligated the funds in fiscal year 1999 based on an appropriation for fiscal year 1998.

Source: Information obtained from departments and agencies.

Appendix III: Examples of Coordination Activities on Bioterrorism Among Federal Departments and Agencies

We identified the following federal departments and agencies as having responsibilities related to the public health and medical consequences of a bioterrorist attack:

- USDA – U.S. Department of Agriculture
  - APHIS – Animal and Plant Health Inspection Service
  - ARS – Agricultural Research Service
  - FSIS – Food Safety Inspection Service
  - OCPM – Office of Crisis Planning and Management
- DOC – Department of Commerce
  - NIST – National Institute of Standards and Technology
- DOD – Department of Defense
  - DARPA – Defense Advanced Research Projects Agency
  - JTFCS – Joint Task Force for Civil Support
  - National Guard
  - U.S. Army
- DOE – Department of Energy
- HHS – Department of Health and Human Services
  - AHRQ – Agency for Healthcare Research and Quality
  - CDC – Centers for Disease Control and Prevention
  - FDA – Food and Drug Administration
  - NIH – National Institutes of Health
  - OEP – Office of Emergency Preparedness
- DOJ – Department of Justice
  - FBI – Federal Bureau of Investigation
  - OJP – Office of Justice Programs
- DOT – Department of Transportation
  - USCG – U.S. Coast Guard
- Treasury – Department of the Treasury
  - USSS – U.S. Secret Service
- VA – Department of Veterans Affairs
- EPA – Environmental Protection Agency
- FEMA – Federal Emergency Management Agency

Figure 1, which is based on the framework given in the Terrorism Incident Annex of the Federal Response Plan, shows a sample of the coordination activities by these federal departments and agencies, as they existed prior to the recent creation of the Office of Homeland Security. This figure illustrates the complex relationships among the many federal departments and agencies involved. The following coordination activities are represented on the figure:

- OMB Oversight of Terrorism Funding. The Office of Management and Budget established a reporting system on the budgeting and expenditure of funds to combat terrorism, with goals to reduce overlap and improve coordination as part of the annual budget cycle.

- Federal Response Plan – Health and Medical Services Annex. This annex to the Federal Response Plan states that HHS is the primary agency for coordinating federal assistance to supplement state and local resources in response to public health and medical care needs in an emergency, including a bioterrorist attack.
- Informal Working Group – Equipment Request Review. This group meets as necessary to review equipment requests of state and local jurisdictions to ensure that duplicative funding is not being given for the same activities.
- Agreement on Tracking Diseases in Animals That Can Be Transmitted to Humans. This group is negotiating an agreement to share information and expertise on tracking diseases that can be transmitted from animals to people and could be used in a bioterrorist attack.
- National Medical Response Team Caches. These caches form a stockpile of drugs for OEP's National Medical Response Teams.
- Domestic Preparedness Program. This program was formed in response to the National Defense Authorization Act of Fiscal Year 1997 (P.L. 104-201) and required DOD to enhance the capability of federal, state, and local emergency responders regarding terrorist incidents involving WMDs and high-yield explosives. As of October 1, 2000, DOD and DOJ share responsibilities under this program.
- Office of National Preparedness – Consequence Management of WMD Attack. In May 2001, the President asked the Director of FEMA to establish this office to coordinate activities of the listed agencies that address consequence management resulting from the use of WMDs.
- Food Safety Surveillance Systems. These systems are FoodNet and PulseNet, two surveillance systems for identifying and characterizing contaminated food.
- National Disaster Medical System. This system, a partnership between federal agencies, state and local governments, and the private sector, is intended to ensure that resources are available to provide medical services following a disaster that overwhelms the local health care resources.
- Collaborative Funding of Smallpox Research. These agencies conduct research on vaccines for smallpox.
- National Pharmaceutical Stockpile Program. This program maintains repositories of life-saving pharmaceuticals, antidotes, and medical supplies that can be delivered to the site of a biological (or other) attack.
- National Response Teams. The teams constitute a national planning, policy, and coordinating body to provide guidance before and assistance during an incident.
- Interagency Group for Equipment Standards. This group develops and maintains a standardized equipment list of essential items for responding to a terrorist WMD attack. (The complete name for this group is the Interagency Board for Equipment Standardization and Interoperability.)
- Force Packages Response Team. This is a grouping of military units that are designated to respond to an incident.
- Cooperative Work on Rapid Detection of Biological Agents in Animals, Plants, and Food. This cooperative group is developing a system to improve on-site rapid detection of biological agents in animals, plants, and food.

Figure 1: Examples of Coordination Activities on Bioterrorism Among Federal Departments and Agencies

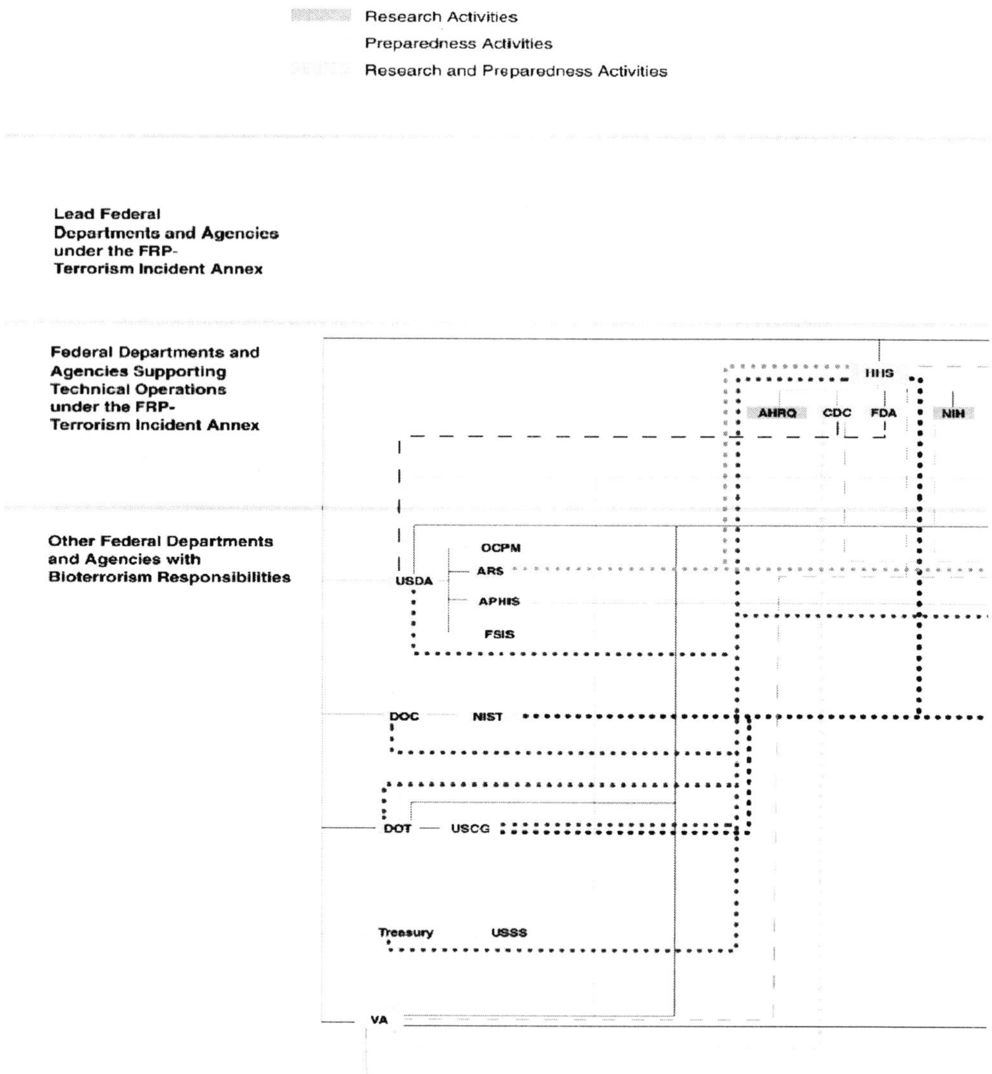

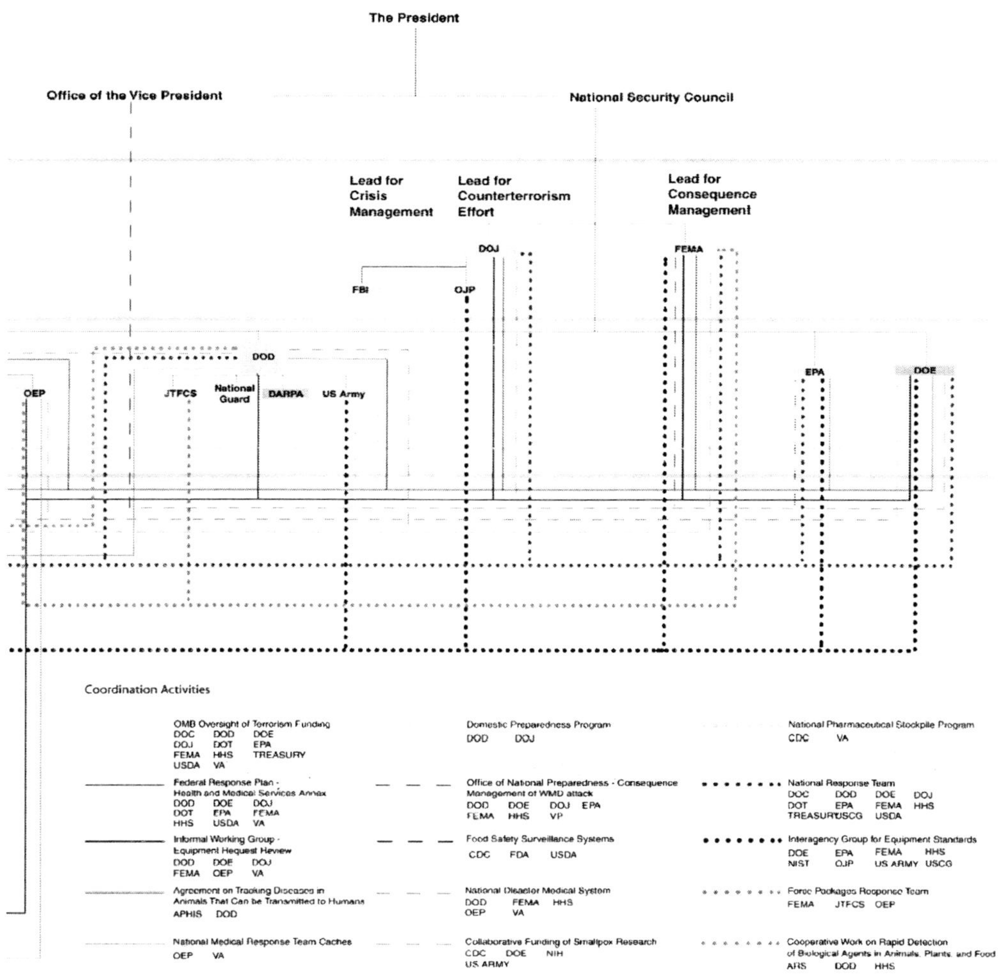
The President
Office of the Vice President
National Security Council
Lead for Crisis Management
Lead for Counterterrorism Effort
Lead for Consequence Management
DOJ
FEMA
FBI
OJP
DOD
OEP
JTFCS
National Guard
DARPA
US Army
EPA
DOE
Coordination Activities
OMB Oversight of Terrorism Funding
DOC DOD DOE
DOJ DOT EPA
FEMA HHS TREASURY
USDA VA
Federal Response Plan - Health and Medical Services Annex
DOD DOE DOJ
DOT EPA FEMA
HHS USDA VA
Informal Working Group - Equipment Request Review
DOD DOE DOJ
FEMA OEP VA
Agreement on Tracking Diseases in Animals That Can be Transmitted to Humans
APHIS DOD
National Medical Response Team Caches
OEP VA
Domestic Preparedness Program
DOD DOJ
Office of National Preparedness - Consequence Management of WMD attack
DOD DOE DOJ EPA
FEMA HHS VP
Food Safety Surveillance Systems
CDC FDA USDA
National Disaster Medical System
DOD FEMA HHS
OEP VA
Collaborative Funding of Smallpox Research
CDC DOE NIH
US ARMY
National Pharmaceutical Stockpile Program
CDC VA
National Response Team
DOC DOD DOE DOJ
DOT EPA FEMA HHS
TREASURY USCG USDA
Interagency Group for Equipment Standards
DOE EPA FEMA HHS
NIST OJP US ARMY USCG
Force Packages Response Team
FEMA JTFCS OEP
Cooperative Work on Rapid Detection of Biological Agents in Animals, Plants, and Food
ARS DOD HHS

Chapter 5

BIOTERRORISM: THE CENTERS FOR DISEASE CONTROL AND PREVENTION'S ROLE IN PUBLIC HEALTH PROTECTION[‡‡]

Janet Heinrich

This chapter discusses the GAO's work on the Centers for Disease Control and Prevention's (CDC) activities to prepare the nation to respond to the public health and medical consequences of a bioterrorist attack.[1] The country is now dealing with anthrax exposures resulting from the agent being sent through the mail and the consequences of dealing with even limited exposures have proven to be quite significant. Prior to the recent anthrax incidents, a domestic bioterrorist attack had been considered to be a low-probability event, in part because of the various difficulties involved in successfully delivering biological agents to achieve large-scale casualties.[2]

On September 28, 2001, we released a report[3] that describes (1) the research and preparedness activities being undertaken by federal departments and agencies to manage the consequences of a bioterrorist attack, (2) the coordination of these activities, and (3) the findings of reports on the preparedness of state and local jurisdictions to respond to a bioterrorist attack. This statement will summarize our findings in the September report

---

‡‡ *Testimony Before the Committee on Energy and Commerce, House of Representatives. November 15, 2001.* Excerpted from GAO Report GAO-02-235T.

[1] Bioterrorism is the threat or intentional release of biological agents (viruses, bacteria, or their toxins) for the purposes of influencing the conduct of government or intimidating or coercing a civilian population.

[2] See *Combating Terrorism: Need for Comprehensive Threat and Risk Assessments of Chemical and Biological Attacks* (GAO/NSIAD-99-163, Sept. 14, 1999), pp. 10-15, for a discussion of the level of difficulty a terrorist would face in attempting to cause mass casualties by making or using chemical or biological agents without the assistance of a state-sponsored program.

[3] See *Bioterrorism: Federal Research and Preparedness Activities* (GAO-01-915, Sept. 28, 2001). This report was mandated by the Public Health Improvement Act of 2000 (P.L. 106-505, sec. 102). We conducted interviews with and obtained information from the Departments of Agriculture, Commerce, Defense, Energy, Health and Human Services (including CDC), Justice, Transportation, the Treasury, and Veterans Affairs; the Environmental Protection Agency; and the Federal Emergency Management Agency.

regarding CDC's research and preparedness activities on bioterrorism and augments our previous work on combating terrorism.[4] Specifically, we will focus on CDC's research and preparedness activities on bioterrorism, and remaining gaps that could hamper the response to a bioterrorist event.

In summary, CDC has a variety of ongoing research and preparedness activities related to bioterrorism. Most of CDC's activities to counter bioterrorism are focused on building and expanding public health infrastructure[5] at the federal, state, and local levels. These include funding research on anthrax and smallpox vaccines, increasing laboratory capacity, and building a national pharmaceutical stockpile of drugs and supplies to be used in an emergency. Since CDC's bioterrorism program began in 1999, funding increased 43 percent in fiscal year 2000 and an additional 12 percent in fiscal year 2001. While the percentage increases are substantial, they reflect only a $73 million increase in overall spending because many of the activities initially received relatively small allocations. Gaps in CDC's activities could hamper the response to a bioterrorist attack. For instance, laboratories at all levels can quickly become overwhelmed with requests for tests. In addition, there is a notable lack of training focused on detecting and responding to bioterrorist threats.

BACKGROUND

Although many aspects of an effective response to bioterrorism are the same as those for any form of terrorism, there are some unique features. For example, if a biological agent is released covertly, it may not be recognized for a week or more because symptoms may not appear for several days after the initial exposure and may be misdiagnosed at first. In addition, some biological agents, such as smallpox, are communicable and can spread to others who were not initially exposed. These characteristics require responses that are unique to bioterrorism, including health surveillance,[6] epidemiologic investigation,[7] laboratory identification of biological agents, and distribution of antibiotics to large segments of the population to prevent the spread of an infectious disease. However, some aspects of an effective response to bioterrorism are also important in responding to any type of large-scale disaster, such as providing emergency medical services, continuing health care services delivery, and, potentially, managing mass fatalities.

The burden of responding to bioterrorist incidents falls initially on personnel in state and local emergency response agencies. These "first responders" include fire-fighters, emergency medical service personnel, law enforcement officers, public health officials, health care workers (including doctors, nurses, and other medical professionals), and public works personnel. If the emergency requires federal disaster assistance, federal departments and agencies will respond according to responsibilities outlined in the Federal Response Plan.[8]

---

[4] See the list of related GAO products at the end of this statement.

[5] The public health infrastructure is the underlying foundation that supports the planning, delivery, and evaluation of public health activities and practices.

[6] Health surveillance systems provide for the ongoing collection, analysis, and dissemination of data to prevent and control disease.

[7] Epidemiological investigation is the study of patterns of health or disease and the factors that influence these patterns.

[8] The Federal Response Plan, originally drafted in 1992 and updated in 1999, is authorized under the Robert T. Stafford Disaster Relief and Emergency Assistance Act (Stafford Act; P.L. 93-288, as amended). The plan

Under the Federal Response Plan, CDC is the lead Department of Health and Human Services (HHS) agency providing assistance to state and local governments for five functions: (1) health surveillance, (2) worker health and safety, (3) radiological, chemical, and biological hazard consultation, (4) public health information, and (5) vector control.[9] Each of these functions is described in table 1.

Table 1: CDC's Functions under the Federal Response Plan

Function	Description of function
Health surveillance	Assist in establishing surveillance systems to monitor the general population and special high-risk population segments; carry out field studies and investigations; monitor injury and disease patterns and potential disease outbreaks; and provide technical assistance and consultations on disease and injury prevention and precautions.
Worker health and safety	Assist in monitoring health and well-being of emergency workers; perform field investigations and studies; and provide technical assistance and consultation on worker health and safety measures and precautions.
Radiological, chemical, and biological hazard consultation	Assist in assessing health and medical effects of radiological, chemical, and biological exposures on the general population and on high-risk population groups; conduct field investigations, including collection and analysis of relevant samples; advise on protective actions related to direct human and animal exposure, and on indirect exposure through radiologically, chemically, or biologically contaminated food, drugs, water supply, and other media; and provide technical assistance and consultation on medical treatment and decontamination of radiologically, chemically, or biologically injured or contaminated victims.
Public health information	Assist by providing public health and disease and injury prevention information that can be transmitted to members of the general public who are located in or near areas affected by a major disaster or emergency.
Vector control	Assist in assessing the threat of vector-borne diseases following a major disaster or emergency; conduct field investigations, including the collection and laboratory analysis of relevant samples; provide vector control equipment and supplies; provide technical assistance and consultation on protective actions regarding vector-borne diseases; and provide technical assistance and consultation on medical treatment of victims of vector-borne diseases.

Source: The Health and Medical Services Annex in the Federal Response Plan, April 1999.

HHS is currently leading an effort to work with governmental and nongovernmental partners to upgrade the nation's public health infrastructure and capacities to respond to

outlines the planning assumptions, policies, concept of operations, organizational structures, and specific assignment of responsibilities to lead departments and agencies in providing federal assistance once the President has declared an emergency requiring federal assistance.

[9] A vector is a carrier, such as an insect, that transmits the organisms of disease from infected to noninfected individuals.

bioterrorism.[10] As part of this effort, several CDC centers, institutes, and offices work together in the agency's Bioterrorism Preparedness and Response Program. The principal priority of CDC's program is to upgrade infrastructure and capacity to respond to a large-scale epidemic, regardless of whether it is the result of a bioterrorist attack or a naturally occurring infectious disease outbreak. The program was started in fiscal year 1999 and was tasked with building and enhancing national, state, and local capacity; developing a national pharmaceutical stockpile; and conducting several independent studies on bioterrorism.

CDC's Research and Preparedness Activities on Bioterrorism

CDC is conducting a variety of activities related to research on and preparedness for a bioterrorist attack. Since CDC's program began 3 years ago, funding for these activities has increased. Research activities focus on detection, treatment, vaccination, and emergency response equipment. Preparedness efforts include increasing state and local response capacity, increasing CDC's response capacity, preparedness and response planning, and building the National Pharmaceutical Stockpile Program.

Trends in CDC's Funding for Bioterrorism Activities

The funding for CDC's activities related to research on and preparedness for a bioterrorist attack has increased 61 percent over the past 2 years. See table 2 for reported funding for these activities.

Funding for CDC's Bioterrorism Preparedness and Response Program grew approximately 43 percent in fiscal year 2000 and an additional 12 percent in fiscal year 2001. While the percentage increases are significant, they reflect only a $73 million increase because many of the programs initially received relatively small allocations. Approximately $45 million of the overall two-year increase was due to new research activities.

Relative changes in funding for the various components of CDC's Bioterrorism Preparedness and Response Program are shown in Figure 1. Funding for research activities increased sharply from fiscal year 1999 to fiscal year 2000, and then dropped slightly in fiscal year 2001. The increase in fiscal year 2000 was largely due to a $40.5 million increase in research funding for studies on anthrax and smallpox. Funding for preparedness and response planning, upgrading CDC capacity, and upgrading state and local capacity was relatively constant between fiscal year 1999 and fiscal year 2000 and grew in fiscal year 2001. For example, funding increased to upgrade CDC capacity by 47 percent and to upgrade state and local capacity by 17 percent in fiscal year 2001. The National Pharmaceutical Stockpile Program experienced a slight increase in funding of 2 percent in fiscal year 2000 and a slight decrease in funding of 2 percent in fiscal year 2001.

[10] Beyond CDC, other offices and agencies within HHS are involved in this effort, including the Agency for Healthcare Research and Quality, the Food and Drug Administration, the National Institutes of Health, and the Office of Emergency Preparedness.

Table 2: Reported Funding for CDC's Bioterrorism Preparedness and Response Program Activities (Dollars in millions)

Program/initiative[a]	Fiscal year 1999	Fiscal year 2000	Fiscal year 2001
Research activities			
Research and development	0	$40.5	$42.9
Independent studies[b]	$1.8	$7.7	$2.6
Worker safety	0	0	$1.1
Preparedness activities			
Upgrading state and local capacity	**$55.0**	**$56.9**	**$66.7**
Preparedness planning	$2.0	$1.9	$5.8
Surveillance and epidemiology	$12.0	$15.8	$16.1
Laboratory capacity	$13.0	$9.5	$12.8
Communications	$28.0	$29.7	$32.0
Upgrading CDC capacity	**$12.0**	**$13.9**	**$20.4**
Epidemiologic capacity	$2.0	$1.8	$4.0
Laboratory capacity	$5.0	$7.6	$11.4
Rapid toxic screening	$5.0	$4.5	$5.0
Preparedness and response planning	$1.0	$2.3	$9.2
Building the National Pharmaceutical Stockpile Program	**$51.0**	**$51.8**	**$51.0**
Total	**$120.8**	**$173.1**	**$193.9**

Note: We have not audited or otherwise verified the information provided.

[a] CDC also received funding in fiscal year 1999, fiscal year 2000, and fiscal year 2001 for bioterrorism deterrence activities, such as implementing regulations restricting the importation of certain biological agents. That funding is not included here.

[b] For instance, $1 million was specified in the fiscal year 2000 appropriations conference report for the Carnegie Mellon Research Institute to study health and bioterrorism threats.

Source: CDC.

Research Activities

CDC's research activities focus on detection, treatment, vaccination, and emergency response equipment. In fiscal year 2001, CDC was allocated $18 million to continue research on an anthrax vaccine and associated issues, such as scheduling and dosage. The agency also received $22.4 million in fiscal year 2001 to conduct smallpox research. In addition, CDC oversees a number of independent studies, which fund specific universities and hospitals to do research and other work on bioterrorism. For example, funding in fiscal year 2001 included $941,000 to the University of Findlay in Findlay, Ohio, to develop training for health care providers and other hospital staff on how to handle victims who come to an emergency department during a bioterrorist incident. Another $750,000 was provided to the University of Texas Medical Branch in Galveston, Texas, to study various viruses in order to discover means to prevent or treat infections by these and other viruses (such as Rift Valley Fever and the smallpox virus). For worker safety, CDC's National Institute for Occupational Safety and Health is developing standards for respiratory protection equipment used against biological agents by firefighters, laboratory technicians, and other potentially affected workers.

Figure 1: CDC's Bioterrorism Preparedness and Response Program Funding

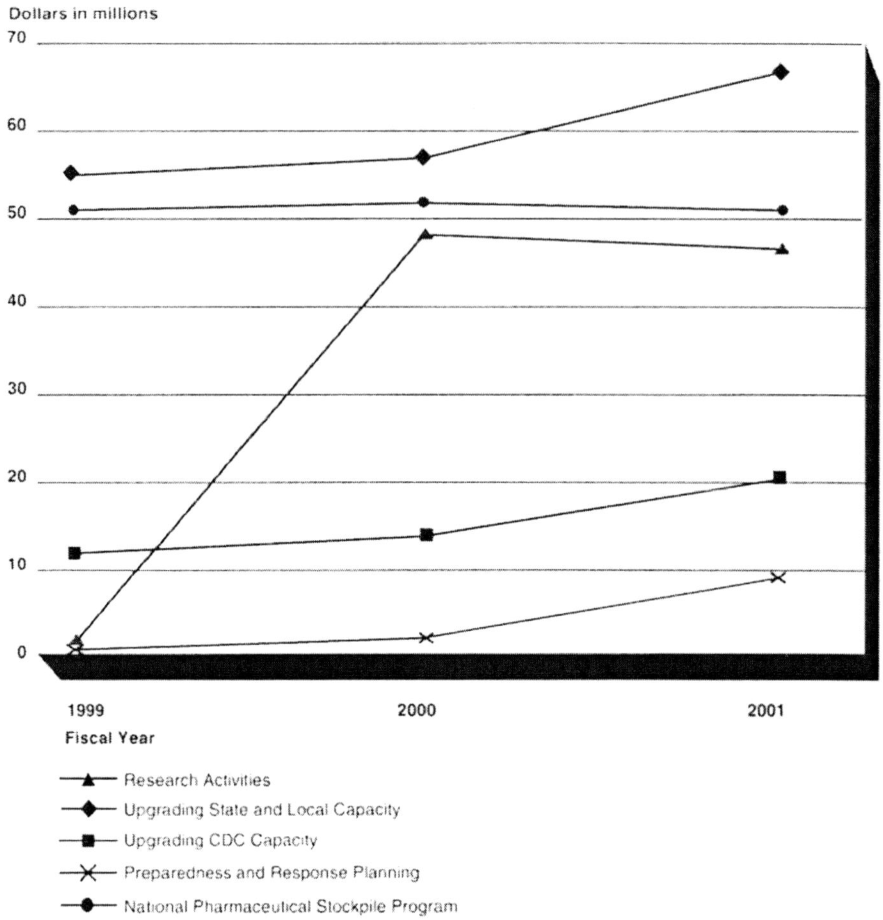

Source: GAO analysis of CDC data.

Preparedness Activities

Most of CDC's activities to counter bioterrorism are focused on building and expanding public health infrastructure at the federal, state, and local levels. For example, CDC reported receiving funding to upgrade state and local capacity to detect and respond to a bioterrorist attack. CDC received additional funding for upgrading its own capacity in these areas, for preparedness and response planning, and for developing the National Pharmaceutical Stockpile Program. In addition to preparing for a bioterrorist attack, these activities also prepare the agency to respond to other challenges, such as identifying and containing a naturally occurring emerging infectious disease.

Upgrading State and Local Capacity

CDC provides grants, technical support, and performance standards to support bioterrorism preparedness and response planning at the state and local levels. In fiscal year 2000, CDC funded 50 states and four major metropolitan health departments for preparedness and response activities. CDC is developing planning guidance for state public health officials to upgrade state and local public health departments' preparedness and response capabilities. In addition, CDC has worked with the Department of Justice to complete a public health assessment tool, which is being used to determine the ability of state and local public health agencies to respond to release of biological and chemical agents, as well as other public health emergencies. Ten states (Florida, Hawaii, Maine, Michigan, Minnesota, Pennsylvania, Rhode Island, South Carolina, Utah, and Wisconsin) have completed the assessment, and others are currently completing it.

States have received funding from CDC to increase staff, enhance capacity to detect the release of a biological agent or an emerging infectious disease, and improve communications infrastructure. In fiscal year 1999, for example, a total of $7.8 million was awarded to 41 state and local health agencies to improve their ability to link different sources of data, such as sales of certain pharmaceuticals, which could be helpful in detecting a covert bioterrorist event.

Rapid identification and confirmatory diagnosis of biological agents are critical to ensuring that prevention and treatment measures can be implemented quickly. CDC was allocated $13 million in fiscal year 1999 to enhance state and local laboratory capacity. CDC has established a Laboratory Response Network of federal, state, and local laboratories that maintain state-of-the-art capabilities for biological agent identification and characterization of human clinical samples such as blood. CDC has provided technical assistance and training in identification techniques to state and local public health laboratories. In addition, five state health departments received awards totaling $3 million to enhance chemical laboratory capabilities from the fiscal year 2000 funds. The states used these funds to purchase equipment and provide training.

CDC is working with state and local health agencies to improve electronic infrastructure for public health communications for the collection and transmission of information related to a bioterrorism incident as well as other events. For example, $21 million was awarded to states in fiscal year 1999 to begin implementation of the Health Alert Network, which will support the exchange of key information over the Internet and provide a means to conduct distance training that could potentially reach a large segment of the public health community. Currently, 13 states are connected to all of their local jurisdictions. CDC is also directly connected to groups such as the American Medical Association to reach healthcare providers.

CDC has described the Health Alert Network as a "highway" on which programs, such as the National Electronic Disease Surveillance System (NEDSS) and the Epidemic Information Exchange (Epi-X), will run. NEDSS is designed to facilitate the development of an integrated, coherent national system for public health surveillance. Ultimately, it is meant to support the automated collection, transmission, and monitoring of disease data from multiple sources (for example, clinician's offices and laboratories) from local to state health departments to CDC. This year, a total of $10.9 million will go to 36 jurisdictions for new or continuing NEDSS activities. Epi-X is a secure, Web-based exchange for public health officials to rapidly report and discuss disease outbreaks and other health events potentially related to bioterrorism as they are identified and investigated.

Upgrading CDC Capacity

CDC is upgrading its own epidemiologic and disease surveillance capacity. It has deployed, and is continuing to enhance, a surveillance system to increase surveillance and epidemiological capacities before, during, and after special events (such as the 1999 World Trade Organization meeting in Seattle). Besides improving emergency response at the special events, the agency gains valuable experience in developing and practicing plans to combat terrorism. In addition, CDC monitors unusual clusters of illnesses, such as influenza in June. Although unusual clusters are not always a cause for concern, they can indicate a potential problem. The agency is also increasing its surveillance of disease outbreaks in animals.

CDC has strengthened its own laboratory capacity. For example, it is developing and validating new diagnostic tests as well as creating agent-specific detection protocols. In collaboration with the Association of Public Health Laboratories and the Department of Defense, CDC has started a secure Web-based network that allows state, local, and other public health laboratories access to guidelines for analyzing biological agents. The site also allows authenticated users to order critical reagents[11] needed in performing laboratory analysis of samples.

The agency has also opened a Rapid Response and Advance Technology Laboratory, which screens samples for the presence of suspicious biological agents and evaluates new technology and protocols for the detection of biological agents. These technology assessments and protocols, as well as reagents and reference samples, are being shared with state and local public health laboratories.

Preparedness and Response Planning

One activity CDC has undertaken is the implementation of a national bioterrorism response training plan. This plan focuses on preparing CDC officials to respond to bioterrorism and includes the development of exercises to assess progress in achieving bioterrorism preparedness at the federal, state, and local levels. The agency is also developing a crisis communications/media response curriculum for bioterrorism, as well as core capabilities guidelines to assist states and localities in their efforts to build comprehensive anti-bioterrorism programs.

CDC has developed a bioterrorism information Web site. This site provides emergency contact information for state and local officials in the event of possible bioterrorism incidents, a list of critical biological and chemical agents, summaries of state and local bioterrorism projects, general information about CDC's bioterrorism initiative, and links to documents on bioterrorism preparedness and response.

The National Pharmaceutical Stockpile Program maintains a repository of life-saving pharmaceuticals, antidotes, and medical supplies, known as 12-Hour Push Packages, that could be used in an emergency, including a bioterrorist attack. The packages can be delivered to the site of a biological (or chemical) attack within 12 hours of deployment for the treatment of civilians. The first emergency use of the National Pharmaceutical Stockpile occurred on September 11, 2001, when in response to the terrorist attack on the World Trade Center, CDC released one of the eight Push Packages.

Building the National Pharmaceutical Stockpile Program

The National Pharmaceutical Stockpile also includes additional antibiotics, antidotes, other drugs, medical equipment, and supplies, known as the Vendor Managed Inventory, that can be delivered within 24 to 36 hours after the appropriate vendors are notified. Deliveries

[11] A reagent is a substance used to detect the presence of another substance.

from the Vendor Managed Inventory can be tailored to an individual incident. The program received \$51.0 million in fiscal year 1999, \$51.8 million in fiscal year 2000, and \$51.0 million in fiscal year 2001. CDC and the Office of Emergency Preparedness (another agency in HHS that also maintains a stockpile of medical supplies) have encouraged state and local representatives to consider stockpile assets in their emergency planning for a biological attack and have trained representatives from state and local authorities in using the stockpile. The stockpile program also provides technical advisers in response to an event to ensure the appropriate and timely transfer of stockpile contents to authorized state representatives.[12] Recently, individuals who may have been exposed to anthrax through the mail have been given antibiotics from the Vendor Managed Inventory.

GAPS IN CDC'S RESEARCH AND PREPAREDNESS ACTIVITIES FOR BIOTERRORISM

While CDC has funded research and preparedness programs for bioterrorism, a great deal of work remains to be done. CDC and HHS have identified gaps in bioterrorism research and preparedness that need to be addressed. In addition, some of our work on naturally occurring diseases also indicates gaps in preparedness that would be important in the event of a bioterrorist attack.

Research Activities

Gaps in research activities center on vaccines and field testing for infectious agents. CDC has reported that it needs to continue the smallpox vaccine development and production contract begun in fiscal year 2000. This includes clinical testing of the vaccine and submitting a licensing application to the Food and Drug Administration for the prevention of smallpox in adults and children.[13] CDC also plans to conduct further studies of the anthrax vaccine. This research will include studies to better understand the immunological response that correlates with protection against inhalation anthrax and risk factors for adverse events as well as investigating modified vaccination schedules that could maintain protection and result in fewer adverse reactions. The agency has also indicated that it needs to continue research in the area of rapid assay tests to allow field diagnosis of a biological or chemical agent.

Preparedness Activities

Gaps remain in all of the areas of preparedness activities under CDC's program. In particular, there are many unmet needs in upgrading state and local capacity to respond to a bioterrorist attack. There are also further needs in upgrading CDC's capacity, preparedness and response planning, and building the National Pharmaceutical Stockpile.

---

[12] For more information on the National Pharmaceutical Stockpile Program, see *Combating Terrorism: Accountability Over Medical Supplies Needs Further Improvement* (GAO-01-463, Mar. 30, 2001).

Upgrading State and Local Capacity

Health officials at many levels have called for CDC to support bioterrorism planning efforts at the state and local level. In a series of regional meetings from May through September 2000 to discuss issues associated with developing comprehensive bioterrorism response plans, state and local officials identified a need for additional federal support of their planning efforts. This includes federal efforts to develop effective written planning guidance for state and local health agencies and to provide on-site assistance that will ensure optimal preparedness and response.

HHS has noted that surveillance capabilities need to be increased. In addition to enhancing traditional state and local capabilities for infectious disease surveillance, HHS has recognized the need to expand surveillance beyond the boundaries of the public health departments. In the department's *FY 2002—FY 2006 Plan for Combating Bioterrorism*, HHS notes that potential sources for data on morbidity trends include 911 emergency calls, reasons for emergency department visits, hospital bed usage, and the purchase of specific products at pharmacies. Improved monitoring of food is also necessary to reduce its vulnerability as an avenue of infection and of terrorism. Other sources beyond public health departments can provide critical information for detection and identification of an outbreak. For example, the 1999 West Nile virus outbreak showed the importance of links with veterinary surveillance.[14] Initially there were two separate investigations: one of sick people, the other of dying birds. Once the two investigations converged, the link was made, and the virus was correctly identified.

HHS has found that state and local laboratories need to continue to upgrade their facilities and equipment. The department has stated that it would be beneficial if research, hospital, and commercial laboratories that have state-of-the-art equipment and well-trained staff were added to the National Laboratory Response Network. Currently, there are 104 laboratories in the network that can provide testing of biological samples for detection and confirmation of biological agents. Based on the 2000 regional meetings, CDC concluded that it needs to continue to support the laboratory network and identify opportunities to include more clinical laboratories to provide additional surge capacity.

CDC also concluded from the 2000 regional meetings that, although it has begun to develop information systems, it needs to continue to enhance these systems to detect and respond to biological and chemical terrorism. HHS has stated that the work that has begun on the Health Alert Network, NEDSS, and Epi-X needs to continue. One aspect of this work is developing, testing, and implementing standards that will permit surveillance data from different systems to be easily shared.

During the West Nile virus outbreak, while a secure electronic communication network was in place at the time of the initial outbreak, not all involved agencies and officials were capable of using it at the same time. For example, because CDC's laboratory was not linked to the New York State network, the New York State Department of Health had to act as an intermediary in sharing CDC's laboratory test results with local health departments. CDC and the New York State Department of Health laboratory databases were not linked to the

---

[13] Previous plans were for 40 million doses of the vaccine to be produced initially, with expected delivery of the first full-scale production lots in 2004. The department now plans to expand and accelerate production significantly.

[14] See *West Nile Virus Outbreak: Lessons for Public Health Preparedness* (GAO/HEHS-00-180, Sept. 11, 2000).

database in New York City, and laboratory results consequently had to be manually entered there. These problems slowed the investigation of the outbreak.

Moreover, we have testified that there is also a notable lack of training focused on detecting and responding to bioterrorist threats.[15] Most physicians and nurses have never seen cases of certain diseases, such as smallpox or plague, and some biological agents initially produce symptoms that can be easily confused with influenza or other, less virulent illnesses, leading to a delay in diagnosis or identification. Medical laboratory personnel require training because they also lack experience in identifying biological agents such as anthrax.

Upgrading CDC Capacity

HHS has stated that epidemiologic capacity at CDC also needs to be improved. A standard system of disease reporting would better enable CDC to monitor disease, track trends, and intervene at the earliest sign of unusual or unexplained illness.

HHS has noted that CDC needs to enhance its in-house laboratory capabilities to deal with likely terrorist agents. CDC plans to develop agent-specific detection and identification protocols for use by the laboratory response network, a research agenda, and guidelines for laboratory management and quality assurance. CDC also plans further development of its Rapid Response and Advanced Technology Laboratory.

As we reported in September 2000, even the West Nile virus outbreak, which was relatively small and occurred in an area with one of the nation's largest local public health agencies, taxed the federal, state, and local laboratory resources. Both the New York State and the CDC laboratories were quickly inundated with requests for tests during the West Nile virus outbreak, and because of the limited capacity at the New York laboratories, the CDC laboratory handled the bulk of the testing. Officials indicated that the CDC laboratory would have been unable to respond to another outbreak, had one occurred at the same time.

Preparedness and Response Planning

CDC plans to work with other agencies in HHS to develop guidance to facilitate preparedness planning and associated investments by local-level medical and public health systems. The department has stated that to the extent that the guidance can help foster uniformity across local efforts with respect to preparedness concepts and structural and operational strategies, this would enable government units to work more effectively together than if each local approach was essentially unique. More generally, CDC has found a need to implement a national strategy for public health preparedness for bioterrorism, and to work with federal, state, and local partners to ensure communication and teamwork in response to a potential bioterrorist incident.

Planning needs to continue for potential naturally occurring epidemics as well. In October 2000, we reported that federal and state influenza pandemic plans are in various stages of completion and do not completely or consistently address key issues surrounding the purchase, distribution, and administration of vaccines and antiviral drugs.[16] At the time of our report, 10 states either had developed or were developing plans using general guidance from CDC, and 19 more states had plans under development. Outstanding issues remained, however, because certain key federal decisions had not been made. For example, HHS had

---

[15] See *Bioterrorism: Review of Public Health Preparedness Programs* (GAO-02-149T, Oct. 12, 2001).

[16] See *Influenza Pandemic: Plan Needed for Federal and State Response* (GAO-01-4, Oct. 27, 2000).

not determined the proportion of vaccines and antiviral drugs to be purchased, distributed, and administered by the public and private sectors or established priorities for which population groups should receive vaccines and antiviral drugs first when supplies are limited. As of July 2001, HHS continued to work on a national plan. As a result, policies may differ among states and between states and the federal government, and in the event of a pandemic, these inconsistencies could contribute to public confusion and weaken the effectiveness of the public health response.

Building the National Pharmaceutical Stockpile

The recent anthrax incidents have focused a great deal of attention on the national pharmaceutical stockpile. Prior to this, in its *FY2002 – FY2006 Plan for Combating Bioterrorism,* HHS had indicated what actions would be necessary regarding the stockpile over the next several years. These included purchasing additional products so that pharmaceuticals were available for treating additional biological agents in fiscal year 2002, and conducting a demonstration project that incorporates the National Guard in planning for receipt, transport, organization, distribution, and dissemination of stockpile supplies in fiscal year 2003. CDC also proposed providing grants to cities in fiscal year 2004 to hire a stockpile program coordinator to help the community develop a comprehensive plan for handling the stockpile and organizing volunteers trained to manage the stockpile during a chemical or biological event. Clearly, these longer range plans are changing, but the need for these activities remains.

Chapter 6

INFECTIOUS DISEASE OUTBREAKS: BIOTERRORISM PREPAREDNESS EFFORTS HAVE IMPROVED PUBLIC HEALTH RESPONSE CAPACITY, BUT GAPS REMAIN**

Janet Heinrich

WHY GAO DID THIS STYDY

Following the bioterrorist events of the fall of 2001, there has been concern that the nation may not be prepared to respond to a major public health threat, such as the current outbreak of Severe Acute Respiratory Syndrome (SARS). Whether a disease outbreak occurs naturally or is due to the intentional release of a harmful biological agent by a terrorist, much of the initial response would occur at the local level, particularly hospitals and their emergency departments. Efforts to plan for worldwide influenza pandemics are useful for understanding public health preparedness for other large-scale outbreaks.

GAO was asked to examine (1) the preparedness of state and local public health agencies and organizations for responding to a large-scale infectious disease outbreak, (2) the preparedness of hospitals for responding to a large-scale infectious disease outbreak, and (3) federal and state efforts to prepare for an influenza pandemic.

WHAT GAO FOUND

The efforts of state and local public health agencies to prepare for a bioterrorist attack have improved the nation's capacity to respond to infectious disease outbreaks and other major public health threats, but gaps in preparedness remain. GAO found workforce shortages and gaps in disease surveillance and laboratory facilities. The level of preparedness varied across cities GAO visited. Jurisdictions that have had multiple prior experiences with public

---

** Highlights of GAO-03-654T, a *Testimony before the Committee on Government Reform, House of Representatives, April 9, 2003.*

health emergencies were generally more prepared than others. GAO found that regional planning was generally lacking between states but that states were developing their own plans for receiving and distributing medical supplies for emergencies, as well as plans for mass vaccinations in the event of a public health emergency.

GAO found that many hospitals lack the capacity to respond to large-scale infectious disease outbreaks. Most hospitals across the country reported participating in basic planning activities for large-scale infectious disease outbreaks and training staff about biological agents. However, most hospitals lack adequate equipment, isolation facilities, and staff to treat a large increase in the number of patients that may result.

Federal and state officials have not finalized plans for responding to pandemic influenza. These plans do not consistently address problems related to the purchase, distribution, and administration of supplies of vaccines and antiviral drugs that may be needed during a pandemic.

Mr. Chairman and Members of the Committee: I appreciate the opportunity to be here today to discuss the work we have done pertaining to the nation's preparedness to manage major public health threats. The initial response to an outbreak of infectious disease would occur at the local level, with support from the state, whether the outbreak was naturally occurring or due to the intentional release of a harmful biological agent by a terrorist. Just as in a bioterrorist attack, a naturally occurring outbreak could involve public health officials in disease surveillance,[1] epidemiologic investigation,[2] health care delivery, and quarantine management. Because of prior worldwide influenza outbreaks—known as pandemics[3]—federal and state agencies have focused special attention on planning how to address such events, and these efforts are useful for understanding public health preparedness for other large-scale outbreaks. The outbreak of Severe Acute Respiratory Syndrome (SARS)[4] has not infected large numbers of individuals in the United States, but it has raised concerns about the nation's preparedness should it, or other infections, reach pandemic proportions.

Following the bioterrorist events of the fall of 2001, Congress expressed concern that the nation may not be prepared to respond to a major public health threat such as a large-scale outbreak of an infectious disease. State and local response agencies and organizations have recognized the need to strengthen their infrastructure and capacity to respond to a bioterrorist attack. The improvements they are making will also strengthen their ability to identify and respond to other major public health threats, including naturally occurring large-scale infectious disease outbreaks.

Planning for a response to bioterrorism and influenza pandemics targets the public health resources essential for a response to other infectious diseases.

---

[1] Disease surveillance uses systems that provide for the ongoing collection, analysis, and dissemination of health-related data to identify, prevent, and control disease.

[2] An epidemiologic investigation seeks to determine how a disease is distributed in a population and the factors that influence or determine this distribution.

[3] Influenza pandemics are worldwide influenza epidemics that can have successive "waves" of disease and last for up to 3 years. Three pandemics occurred in the twentieth century: the "Spanish flu" of 1918, which killed at least 20 million people worldwide; the "Asian flu" of 1957; and the "Hong Kong flu" of 1968.

[4] SARS is a respiratory illness that has recently been reported principally in Asia, Europe, and North America. As of April 7, 2003, there were an estimated 2,601 cases reported in 19 countries, including 141 suspected cases in the United States. There have been 98 deaths worldwide, none of which have been in the United States. Symptoms of the disease, which may be caused by a previously unrecognized coronavirus, can include a fever, chills, headache, other body aches, or a dry cough.

To assist the Committee in its consideration of our nation's capacity to respond to a major public health threat, my remarks today will focus on (1) the preparedness of state and local public health agencies for responding to a large-scale infectious disease outbreak, (2) the preparedness of hospitals for responding to a large-scale infectious disease outbreak, and (3) federal and state efforts to prepare for an influenza pandemic.

My testimony today is based largely on our recently released report on state and local preparedness for a bioterrorist attack.[5] For that report, we conducted site visits to seven cities and their respective state governments. We also reviewed each state's spring 2002 applications for bioterrorism preparedness funding distributed by the Department of Health and Human Services' (HHS) Centers for Disease Control and Prevention (CDC) and Health Resources and Services Administration (HRSA), and each state's fall 2002 progress report on the use of that funding. In addition, I will present some initial findings from a survey we conducted of hospitals to assess their level of emergency preparedness, which we will more fully report later, and from information updating our 2000 report on federal and state planning for an influenza pandemic.[6]

In summary, while the efforts of public health agencies and health care organizations to prepare for a bioterrorist attack have improved the nation's capacity to respond to infectious disease outbreaks and other major public health threats, gaps in preparedness remain. More specifically, we found that there are gaps in disease surveillance systems and laboratory facilities, and that there are workforce shortages. The level of preparedness varied across cities we visited, with jurisdictions that have had multiple prior experiences with public health emergencies being generally more prepared than others. We found that regional planning was lacking between states, but states were developing their own plans for receiving and distributing medical supplies for emergencies, and for mass vaccinations in the event of a public health emergency. We found that many hospitals lack the capacity to respond to large-scale infectious disease outbreaks. Although most hospitals across the country report participating in basic planning activities for such outbreaks, few have adequate medical equipment, such as ventilators, needed to handle the large increases in the number of patients that may result. Federal and state influenza pandemic response plans, another component of public health preparedness, are in various stages of completion and do not consistently address the problems related to the purchase, distribution, and administration of supplies of vaccines and antiviral drugs during a pandemic.

BACKGROUND

In order to be adequately prepared for a major public health threat, state and local public health agencies need to have several basic capabilities, whether they possess them directly or have access to them through regional agreements. Public health departments need to have disease surveillance systems and epidemiologists to detect clusters of suspicious symptoms or diseases in order to facilitate early detection of disease and treatment of victims. Laboratories need to have adequate capacity and necessary staff to test clinical and environmental samples

[5] U.S. General Accounting Office, *Bioterrorism: Preparedness Varied across State and Local Jurisdictions*, GAO-03-373 (Washington, D.C.: Apr. 7, 2003).

[6] U.S. General Accounting Office, *Influenza Pandemic: Plan Needed for Federal and State Response*, GAO-01-4 (Washington, D.C.: Oct. 27, 2000).

in order to identify an agent promptly so that proper treatment can be started and infectious diseases prevented from spreading. All organizations involved in the response must be able to communicate easily with one another as events unfold and critical information is acquired, especially in a large-scale infectious disease outbreak. In addition, plans that describe how state and local officials would manage and coordinate an emergency response need to be in place and to have been tested in an exercise, both at the state and local levels as well as at the regional level.

Local health care organizations, including hospitals, are generally responsible for the initial response to a public health emergency, be it a bioterrorist attack or a naturally occurring infectious disease outbreak. In the event of a large-scale infectious disease outbreak, hospitals and their emergency departments would be on the front line, and their personnel would take on the role of first responders. Because hospital emergency departments are open 24 hours a day, 7 days a week, exposed individuals would be likely to seek treatment from the medical staff on duty. Staff would need to be able to recognize and report any illness patterns or diagnostic clues that might indicate an unusual infectious disease outbreak to their state or local health department. Hospitals would need to have the capacity and staff necessary to treat severely ill patients and limit the spread of infectious disease. In addition, hospitals would need adequate stores of equipment and supplies, including medications, personal protective equipment, quarantine and isolation facilities, and air handling and filtration equipment.

The federal government also has a role in preparedness for and response to major public health threats. It becomes involved in investigating the cause of the disease, as it is doing with SARS. In addition, the federal government provides funding and resources to state and local entities to support preparedness and response efforts. CDC's Public Health Preparedness and Response for Bioterrorism program provided funding through cooperative agreements in fiscal year 2002 totaling $918 million to states and municipalities to improve bioterrorism preparedness and response, as well as other public health emergency preparedness activities. HRSA's Bioterrorism Hospital Preparedness Program provided funding through cooperative agreements in fiscal year 2002 of approximately $125 million to states and municipalities to enhance the capacity of hospitals and associated health care entities to respond to bioterrorist attacks. Among the other public health emergency response resources that the federal government provides is the Strategic National Stockpile, which contains pharmaceuticals, antidotes, and medical supplies that can be delivered anywhere in the United States within 12 hours of the decision to deploy.

Officials view influenza vaccine as the cornerstone of efforts to prevent and control annual influenza outbreaks as well as pandemic influenza. Deciding which viral strains to include in the annual influenza vaccine depends on data collected from domestic and international surveillance systems that identify prevalent strains and characterize their effect on human health.[7] Antiviral drugs and vaccines against influenza are expected to be in short supply if a pandemic occurs. Antiviral drugs, which can be used against all forms of viral diseases, have been as effective as vaccines in preventing illness from influenza and have the advantage of being available now. HHS assumes shortages will occur in a pandemic because

[7] CDC participates in international disease and laboratory surveillance sponsored by the World Health Organization, which operates in 83 countries.

demand is expected to exceed current rates of production and increasing production capacity of antiviral drugs can take at least 6 to 9 months, according to manufacturers.

State and Local Officials Reported Varying Levels of Public Health Preparedness for Infectious Diseases Outbreaks

In the cities we visited, state and local officials reported varying levels of public health preparedness to respond to an infectious disease outbreak. They recognized gaps in preparedness elements such as communication and were beginning to address them. Gaps also remained in other preparedness elements that have been more difficult to address, including the response capacity of the workforce and the disease surveillance and laboratory systems. In addition, we found that the level of preparedness varied across the cities. Jurisdictions that had multiple prior experiences with public health emergencies were generally more prepared than those with little or no such experience prior to our site visits. We found that regional planning was lacking between states. States were working on their own plans for receiving and distributing the Strategic National Stockpile and for administering mass vaccinations.

Progress Has Been Made in Elements of Public Health Preparedness, But Gaps Remain

States and local areas were addressing gaps in public health preparedness elements, such as communication, but weaknesses remained in other preparedness elements, including the response capacity of the workforce and the disease surveillance and laboratory systems. Gaps in capacity often are not amenable to solution in the short term because either they require additional resources or the solution takes time to implement.

Communication

We found that officials were beginning to address communication problems. For example, six of the seven cities we visited were examining how communication would take place in a public health emergency. Many cities had purchased communication systems that allow officials from different organizations to communicate with one another in real time. In addition, state and local health agencies were working with CDC to build the Health Alert Network (HAN), an information and communication system. The nationwide HAN program has provided funding to establish infrastructure at the local level to improve the collection and transmission of information related to public health preparedness, including preparedness for a bioterrorism incident. Goals of the HAN program include providing high-speed Internet connectivity, broadcast capacity for emergency communication, and distance-learning infrastructure for training.

Surveillance Systems and Laboratory Facilities

State and local officials for the cities we visited recognized and were attempting to address inadequacies in their surveillance systems and laboratory facilities. Local officials were concerned that their surveillance systems were inadequate to detect a bioterrorist event and all of the states we visited were making efforts to improve their disease surveillance systems. Six of the cities we visited used a passive surveillance system[8] to detect infectious disease outbreaks.[9] However, passive systems may be inadequate to identify a rapidly spreading outbreak in its earliest and most manageable stage because, as officials in three states noted, there is chronic underreporting and a time lag between diagnosis of a condition and the health department's receipt of the report. To improve disease surveillance, six of the states and two of the cities we visited were developing surveillance systems using electronic databases. Several cities were also evaluating the use of nontraditional data sources, such as pharmacy sales, to conduct surveillance.[10] Three of the cities we visited were attempting to improve their surveillance capabilities by incorporating active surveillance components into their systems.

However, work to improve surveillance systems has proved challenging. For example, despite initiatives to develop active surveillance systems, the officials in one city considered event detection to be a weakness in their system, in part because they did not have authority to access hospital information systems. In addition, various local public health officials in other cities reported that they lacked the resources to sustain active surveillance.

Officials from all of the states we visited reported problems with their public health laboratory systems and said that they needed to be upgraded. All states were planning to purchase the equipment necessary for rapidly identifying a biological agent. State and local officials in most of the areas that we visited told us that the public health laboratory systems in their states were stressed, in some cases severely, by the sudden and significant increases in workload during the anthrax incidents in the fall 2001. During these incidents, the demand for laboratory testing was significant even in states where no anthrax was found and affected the ability of the laboratories to perform their routine public health functions. Following the incidents, over 70,000 suspected anthrax samples were tested in laboratories across the country.

Officials in the states we visited were working on other solutions to their laboratory problems. States were examining various ways to manage peak loads, including entering into agreements with other states to provide surge capacity, incorporating clinical laboratories into cooperative laboratory systems, and purchasing new equipment. One state was working to

---

[8] Passive surveillance systems rely on laboratory and hospital staff, physicians, and other relevant sources to take the initiative to provide data on illnesses to the health department, where officials analyze and interpret the information as it arrives. In contrast, in an active disease surveillance system, public health officials contact sources, such as laboratories, hospitals, and physicians, to obtain information on conditions or diseases in order to identify cases. Active surveillance can provide more complete detection of disease patterns than a system that is wholly dependent on voluntary reporting.

[9] Officials in one city told us that although it had no local disease surveillance, its state maintained a passive disease surveillance system.

[10] This type of active surveillance system in which the public health department obtains information from such sources as hospitals and pharmacies and conducts ongoing analysis of the data to search for certain combinations of signs and symptoms, is sometimes referred to as a syndromic surveillance system. One federal official has stated that research examining the usefulness of syndromic surveillance needs to continue. See S. Lillibridge, `Disease Surveillance, Bioterrorism, and Homeland Security,`

alleviate its laboratory problems by upgrading two local public health laboratories to enable them to process samples of more dangerous pathogens, and establishing agreements with other states to provide backup capacity. Another state reported that it was using the funding from CDC to increase the number of pathogens the state laboratory could diagnose. The state also reported that it has worked to identify laboratories in adjacent states that are capable of being reached within 3 hours over surface roads. In addition, all of the states reported that their laboratory response plans were revised to cover reporting and sharing laboratory results with local public health and law enforcement agencies.

Workforce

At the time of our site visits, shortages in personnel existed in state and local public health departments and laboratories and were difficult to remedy. Officials from state and local health departments told us that staffing shortages were a major concern. Two of the states and cities that we visited were particularly concerned that they did not have enough epidemiologists to do the appropriate investigations in an emergency. One state department of public health we visited had lost approximately one-third of its staff because of budget cuts over the past decade. This department had been attempting to hire more epidemiologists. Barriers to finding and hiring epidemiologists included noncompetitive salaries and a general shortage of people with the necessary skills.

Shortages in laboratory personnel were also cited. Officials in one city noted that they had difficulty filling and maintaining laboratory positions. People that accepted the positions often left the health department for better-paying positions. Increased funding for hiring staff cannot necessarily solve these shortages in the near term because for many types of laboratory positions there are not enough trained individuals in the workforce. According to the Association of Public Health Laboratories, training laboratory personnel to provide them with the necessary skills will take time and require a strategy for building the needed workforce.[11]

Level of Preparedness Varied across Cities We Visited

We found that the overall level of public health preparedness varied by city. In the cities we visited, we observed that those cities that had recurring experience with public health emergencies, including those resulting from natural disasters, or with preparation for National Security Special Events, such as political conventions,[12] were generally more prepared than cities with little or no such experience. Cities that had dealt with multiple public health emergencies in the past might have been further along because they had learned which organizations and officials need to be involved in preparedness and response efforts and moved to include all pertinent parties in the efforts. Experience with natural disasters raised

Conference Summary and Proceedings Prepared by the Annapolis Center for Science-Based Public Policy (Annapolis, Md.: U.S. Medicine Institute for Health Studies, Dec. 4, 2001).

[11] Association of Public Health Laboratories, "State Public Health Laboratory Bioterrorism Capacity," *Public Health Laboratory Issues in Brief: Bioterrorism Capacity* (Washington, D.C.: October 2002).

[12] Presidential Decision Directive 62 created a category of special events called National Security Special Events, which are events of such significance that they warrant greater federal planning and protection than other special events. In addition to major political party conventions, such events include presidential inaugurations.

the awareness of local officials regarding the level of public health emergency preparedness in their cities and the kinds of preparedness problems they needed to address.

Even the cities that were better prepared were not strong in all elements. For example, one city reported that communications had been effective during public health emergencies and that the city had an active disease surveillance system. However, officials reported gaps in laboratory capacity. Another one of the better-prepared cities was connected to HAN and the Epidemic Information Exchange (Epi-X),[13] and all county emergency management agencies in the state were linked. However, the state did not have written agreements with its neighboring states for responding to a public health emergency.

Regional Planning Was Lacking between States

Response organization officials were concerned about a lack of planning for regional coordination between states of the public health response to an infectious disease outbreak. As called for by the guidance for the CDC and HRSA funding, all of the states we visited organized their planning on the basis of regions within their states, assigning local areas to particular regions for planning purposes. A concern for response organization officials was the lack of planning for regional coordination between states. A hospital official in one city we visited said that state lines presented a "real wall" for planning purposes. Hospital officials in one state reported that they had no agreements with other states to share physicians. However, one local official reported that he had been discussing these issues and had drafted mutual aid agreements for hospitals and emergency medical services. Public health officials from several states reported developing working relationships with officials from other states to provide backup laboratory capacity.

States Have Begun Planning for Receiving and Distributing the Strategic National Stockpile and for Administering Mass Vaccinations

States have begun planning for use of the Strategic National Stockpile. To determine eligibility for the CDC funding, applicants were required to develop interim plans to receive and manage items from the stockpile, including mass distribution of antibiotics, vaccines, and medical materiel. However, having plans for the acceptance of the deliveries from the stockpile is not enough. Plans have to include details about dividing the materials that are delivered in large pallets and distributing the medications and vaccines.

Of the seven states we visited, five states had completed plans for the receipt and distribution of the stockpile. One state that was working on its plan stated that it would be completed in January 2003. Only one state had conducted exercises of its stockpile distribution plan, while the other states were planning to conduct exercises or drills of their plans sometime in 2003.

In addition, five states reported on their plans for mass vaccinations and seven states reported on their plans for large-scale administration of smallpox vaccine in response to an outbreak. Some states we visited had completed plans for mass vaccinations, whereas other

---

[13] Epi-X is a secure, Web-based exchange for public health officials to rapidly exchange information on disease outbreaks, exposures to environmental hazards, and other health events as they are identified and investigated.

states were still developing their plans. The mass vaccination plans were generally closely tied to the plans for receiving and administering the stockpile. In addition, two states had completed smallpox response plans, which include administering mass smallpox vaccinations to the general population, whereas four of the other states were drafting plans. The remaining state was discussing such a plan. However, only one of the states we visited has tested in an exercise its plan for conducting mass smallpox vaccinations.

MOST HOSPITALS LACK RESPONSE CAPACITY FOR LARGE-SCALE INFECTIOUS DISEASE OUTBREAKS

Our recent work shows that progress in improving public health response capacity has lagged in hospitals. Although most hospitals across the country reported participating in basic planning activities for large-scale infectious disease outbreaks, few have acquired the medical equipment resources, such as ventilators, to handle large increases in the number of patients that may result from outbreaks of diseases such as SARS.

Most Hospitals Reported Planning and Training Efforts, but Fewer Than Half Have Participated in Drills or Exercises

At the time of our site visits, we found that hospitals were beginning to coordinate with other local response organizations and collaborate with each other in local planning efforts. Hospital officials in one city we visited told us that until September 11, 2001, hospitals were not seen as part of a response to a terrorist event but that the city had come to realize that the first responders to a bioterrorism incident could be a hospital's medical staff. Officials from the state began to emphasize the need for a local approach to hospital preparedness. They said, however, that it was difficult to impress the importance of cooperation on hospitals because hospitals had not seen themselves as part of a local response system. The local government officials were asking them to create plans that integrated the city's hospitals and addressed such issues as off-site triage of patients and off-site acute care.

According to our survey of over 2,000 hospitals,[14] 4 out of 5 hospitals reported having a written emergency response plan for large-scale infectious disease outbreaks. Of these hospitals with emergency response plans, most include a description of how to achieve surge capacity for obtaining additional pharmaceuticals, other supplies, and staff. Almost all hospitals reported participating in community interagency disaster preparedness committees.

Our survey showed that hospitals have provided training to staff on biological agents, but fewer than half have participated in exercises. Most hospitals we surveyed reported providing training about identifying and diagnosing symptoms for the six biological agents identified by

---

[14] Between June and September 2002, we surveyed over 2,000 nonfederal, short-term, general, medical, adult and children's hospitals with emergency departments located in metropolitan statistical areas (see U.S. General Accounting Office, *Hospital Emergency Department: Crowded Conditions Vary among Hospitals and Communities,* GAO-03-460 (Washington, D.C.: Mar. 14, 2003) for information on the survey universe and development of the survey). The survey contained three parts, the third of which specifically addressed hospital preparedness for mass casualty incidents. We obtained responses from 1,482 hospitals for the third section of the survey addressing emergency preparedness, a response rate of about 73 percent.

the CDC as most likely to be used in a bioterrorist attack. While at least 90 percent of hospitals reported providing training for smallpox and anthrax, approximately three-fourths of hospitals reported providing training about plague, botulism, tularemia, and hemorrhagic fever viruses. Fewer than half the hospitals reported participating in drills or exercises related to bioterrorism.

Most Hospitals Lack Adequate Equipment, Facilities, and Staff Required to Respond to a Large-Scale Infectious Disease Outbreak

Most hospitals lack adequate equipment, isolation facilities, and staff to treat a large increase in the number of patients for an infectious disease such as SARS. To prevent transmission of SARS in health care settings, CDC recommends that health care workers use personal protective equipment, including gowns, gloves, respirators, and protective eyewear.[15] SARS patients in the United States are being isolated until they are no longer infectious. CDC estimates that patients require mechanical ventilation in 10 to 20 percent of SARS cases.[16]

In the seven cities we visited, hospital, state, and local officials reported that hospitals needed additional equipment and capital improvements—including medical stockpiles, personal protective equipment, quarantine and isolation facilities, and air handling and filtering equipment—to enhance preparedness. Five of the states we visited reported shortages of hospital medical staff, including nurses and physicians, necessary to increase response capacity in an emergency. One of the states we visited reported that only 11 percent of its hospitals could readily increase their capacity for treating patients with infectious diseases requiring isolation, such as smallpox and SARS. Another state reported that most of its hospitals have little or no capacity for isolating patients diagnosed with or being tested for infectious diseases.

According to our hospital survey, availability of medical equipment varied greatly between hospitals, and few hospitals seemed to have adequate equipment and supplies to handle a large-scale infectious disease outbreak. While most hospitals had at least 1 ventilator per 100 staffed beds, 1 personal protective equipment suit per 100 staffed beds, or an isolation bed per 100 staffed beds, half of the hospitals had less than 6 ventilators per 100 staffed beds, 3 or fewer personal protective equipment suits per 100 staffed beds, and less than 4 isolation beds per 100 staffed beds.

---

15 CDC, *Interim Domestic Guidance for Management of Exposures to Severe Acute Respiratory Syndrome (SARS) for Healthcare and Other Institutional Settings* (Mar. 27, 2003), http://www.cdc.gov/ncidod/sars/exposureguidance.htm (downloaded Apr. 5, 2003).

16 CDC, *SARS Frequently Asked Questions*, http://www.cdc.gov/ncidod/sars/faq.htm (downloaded Apr. 5, 2003).

OFFICIALS HAVE BEEN SLOW TO FINALIZE PLANS FOR FEDERAL AND STATE RESPONSE TO AN INFLUENZA PANDEMIC

Federal and state influenza pandemic response plans, another important component to public health preparedness, are in various stages of completion and do not consistently address the problems related to the purchase, distribution, and administration of supplies of vaccines and antiviral drugs during a pandemic. CDC has provided interim draft guidance to facilitate state plans, but final federal decisions necessary to mitigate the effects of potential shortages of vaccines and antiviral drugs have not been made. Until such decisions are made, the timeliness and adequacy of response efforts may be compromised.

Federal and State Pandemic Response Plans Are Not Finalized

Federal and state officials have not finalized plans for responding to pandemic influenza. To foster state and local pandemic planning and preparedness, CDC first issued interim planning guidance in draft form to all states in 1997, outlining general federal and state planning responsibilities. Thirty-four states are actively preparing a pandemic response plan, and many are integrating these plans with existing state plans to respond to natural or man-made disasters, such as floods or a bioterrorist attack. Although to a certain extent planning efforts for other emergencies can be used for pandemic response, additional planning is important to deal with specific aspects of a pandemic response. This includes developing plans to address the large-scale emergency needs of an entire population, including mass distribution and administration of limited vaccines and drugs, with an uncertain amount of available resources.

Key Federal Decisions Are Unresolved

In the most recent version of its pandemic influenza planning guidance for states, CDC lists several key federal decisions related to vaccines and antiviral drugs that have not been made. These decisions include determining the amount of vaccines and antiviral drugs that will be purchased at the federal level; the division of responsibility between the public and private sectors for the purchase, distribution, and administration of vaccines and drugs; and how population groups will be prioritized and targeted to receive limited supplies of vaccines and drugs. In each of these areas, until federal decisions are made, states will not be able to develop strategies consistent with federal action.

The interim draft guidance for state pandemic plans says that resources can be expected to be available through federal contracts to purchase influenza vaccine and some antiviral agents, but some state funding may be required. The amounts of antiviral drugs to be purchased and stockpiled are yet to be determined, even though these drugs are available and can theoretically be used for both treatment and prevention during a pandemic.

CDC has indicated in its interim draft guidance that the policies for purchasing, distributing, and administering vaccines and drugs by the private and public sector will change during a pandemic, but some decisions necessary to prepare for these expected changes have not been made. During a typical annual influenza response, influenza vaccine and antiviral drug distribution is primarily handled directly by manufacturers through private vendors and pharmacies to health care providers. During a pandemic, however, CDC interim draft guidance indicates that many of these private-sector responsibilities may be transferred to the public sector at the federal, state, or local levels, and priority groups within the population would need to be established for receiving limited supplies of vaccines and drugs.

State officials are particularly concerned that a national plan has not been issued with final recommendations for how population groups should be prioritized to receive vaccines and antiviral drugs. In its interim draft guidance, CDC lists eight population groups that should be considered in establishing priorities among groups for receiving vaccines and drugs during a pandemic. The list includes such groups as health care workers and public health personnel involved in the pandemic response, persons traditionally considered to be at increased risk of severe influenza illness and mortality, and preschool and school-aged children.

Although state officials acknowledge the need for flexibility in planning because many aspects of a pandemic cannot be known in advance, the absence of more detail leaves them uncertain about how to plan for the use of limited supplies of vaccine and drugs. In our 2000 report on the influenza pandemic, we recommended that HHS determine the capability of the private and public sectors to produce, distribute, and administer vaccines and drugs and complete the national response plan.[17] To date, only limited progress has been made in addressing these recommendations.

CONCLUDING OBSERVATIONS

Many actions taken at the state and local level to prepare for a bioterrorist event have enhanced the ability of state and local response agencies and organizations to manage a major public health threat, such as a large-scale infectious disease outbreak. However, there are significant gaps in public health surveillance systems and laboratory capacity, and the number of personnel trained for disease detection is insufficient. Hospitals have begun planning and training efforts to respond to large-scale infectious disease outbreaks, but lack adequate equipment, medical stockpiles, personal protective equipment, and quarantine and isolation facilities. Federal and state plans for the purchase, distribution, and administration of supplies of vaccines and drugs in response to an influenza pandemic have still not been finalized. The lack of these final plans has serious implications for efforts to mobilize the distribution of vaccines and drugs for other infectious disease outbreaks.

[17] GAO-01-4.

Chapter 7

BIOTERRORISM: PUBLIC HEALTH RESPONSE TO ANTHRAX INCIDENTS OF 2001[§]

Janet Heinrich

INTRODUCTION

In the fall of 2001, letters containing anthrax spores were mailed to news media personnel and congressional officials, leading to the first cases of anthrax infection related to an intentional release of anthrax in the United States.[1] Outbreaks of the disease were concentrated in six locations, or epicenters, in the country—Florida; New York; New Jersey; Capitol Hill in Washington, D.C.;[2] the Washington, D.C., regional area, which includes Maryland and Virginia; and Connecticut—where individuals came into contact with spores from the contaminated letters. The anthrax incidents caused illness in 22 people, 11 with the cutaneous (skin) form of the disease and 11 with the inhalational (respiratory) form. Five people died, all from inhalational anthrax. The anthrax incidents and the illness and deaths they caused also had an impact on the country beyond the six epicenters. Across the nation, even in areas far removed from the epicenters, residents brought samples of suspicious powders to officials for testing and worried about the safety of their daily mail.

The public health response to the anthrax incidents was complicated by several factors. The incidents occurred in the turbulent period following the terrorist attacks of September 11, 2001, when the focus of the nation was centered on response to those events. In addition, the anthrax incidents were unprecedented. The response was coordinated by the Department of

---

§ Highlights of GAO-04-152. *A report to the Honorable Bill Frist, Majority Leader, U.S. Senate. October 15, 2003.*

1 Anthrax is a serious disease caused by *Bacillus anthracis*, a bacterium that forms spores. A bacterium is a very small organism made up of one cell. A spore is a dormant bacterium cell that can be revived under certain conditions.

2 In this report, we identify Capitol Hill, the complex of congressional office buildings centering on the U.S. Capitol, as an epicenter distinct from the Washington, D.C., regional area epicenter because Capitol Hill functions independently from the District of Columbia. The Office of the Attending Physician, U.S. Congress, which is an office of the U.S. Navy, serves as the local health department for Capitol Hill and is responsible for the health of about 30,000 public officials and staff, as well as tourists, on Capitol Hill.

Health and Human Services (HHS), primarily through its Centers for Disease Control and Prevention (CDC), and CDC had never responded simultaneously to multiple disease outbreaks caused by the intentional release of an infectious agent. Anthrax was virtually unknown in clinical practice, and many clinicians did not have a good understanding of how to diagnose and treat it. As a result, public health officials at the federal, state, and local levels were basing their actions and recommendations to government officials, other responders,[3] and the public on information that was changing rapidly. The response to the incidents has been characterized by several public officials, academics, and other commentators as problematic and an indication that the country was unprepared for a bioterrorist event.

An examination of the response to the anthrax incidents provides an important opportunity to apply lessons learned from that experience to enhance the nation's preparedness for bioterrorism and other public health emergencies. Because of your interest in bioterrorism preparedness, you asked us to review the public health response to the anthrax incidents. Specifically, you asked us to determine (1) what was learned from the experience that could help improve public health preparedness for bioterrorism at the local and state levels and (2) what was learned that could help improve public health preparedness for bioterrorism at the federal level and what steps have been taken to make those improvements.

In studying the response of local and state public health departments, we interviewed officials from the six epicenters. For a previous report,[4] we had conducted interviews about bioterrorism preparedness with officials from seven cities and their respective state capitals. These interviews were conducted from December 2001 through March 2002, and we used information from these interviews to examine the public health response to the anthrax incidents in localities that were not epicenters. To study federal public health efforts, we interviewed officials from the Department of Defense (DOD) and HHS. These officials included representatives from DOD's Armed Forces Institute of Pathology, Chemical Biological Incident Response Force, Naval Medical Research Center, and U.S. Army Medical Research Institute of Infectious Diseases (USAMRIID), and from HHS's Agency for Healthcare Research and Quality (AHRQ), CDC, Food and Drug Administration (FDA), National Institutes of Health (NIH), and Office of the Assistant Secretary for Public Health Emergency Preparedness. To determine the nature of the information provided by CDC during the incidents, we examined the materials that CDC disseminated during October 2001 through December 2001. For overall assessments of and information on the local, state, and federal public health response, we interviewed members of the academic community and officials of private organizations representing groups affected by the incidents or involved in the response, including the American Hospital Association, the American Medical Association, the American Nurses Association, the American Postal Workers Union, the American Public Health Association, and the District of Columbia Hospital Association. We also reviewed media reports of the incidents from television news services and newspapers, retrospective analyses of the response published after the incidents, relevant congressional hearings that were held between October 2001 and December 2001, and materials provided to us by local, state, and federal agencies and private organizations involved in responding to the

[3] In this report, the term responder refers to any organization or individual that would respond to a bioterrorist incident. These include physicians, nurses, hospitals, laboratories, public health departments, emergency medical services, emergency management agencies, fire departments, and law enforcement agencies.

[4] U.S. General Accounting Office, *Bioterrorism: Preparedness Varied across State and Local Jurisdictions*, GAO-03-373 (Washington, D.C.: Apr. 7, 2003).

attack. To understand the scientific community's analysis of the anthrax incidents, we searched the scientific literature using the National Library of Medicine's PubMed service and reviewed relevant articles. To determine what was learned from the experience that could help improve public health preparedness for bioterrorism, we analyzed these materials for common themes. We focused on what could be learned from the anthrax incidents that could help improve public health preparedness not specifically for anthrax or any particular locality but for bioterrorism in general. To determine what steps have been taken to make those improvements, we reviewed materials from relevant federal agencies through October 2003. Although efforts to decontaminate affected facilities are part of the public health response, they are outside the scope of this report, as is the criminal investigation associated with the incidents.[5] We conducted our work from May 2003 through October 2003 in accordance with generally accepted government auditing standards.

RESULTS IN BRIEF

Local and state public health officials identified strengths in their responses to the anthrax incidents of 2001 as well as areas for improvement. These officials said that their planning efforts had helped to promote a rapid and coordinated response, but they had not fully anticipated the extent of coordination that would be needed across both public and private entities involved in the response to the anthrax incidents. Even though many aspects of their existing response plans had been made operational, for example, by putting agreements into place, the aspects that had not been operationalized affected their ability to coordinate a rapid response to the anthrax incidents. Local and state officials said that their responses also benefited from previous experiences, whether gained through exercising their plans or by responding to emergencies of various kinds. These experiences had allowed them to build relationships and identify areas for improvement in their plans and thus to be better prepared to respond to the anthrax incidents. Local and state officials also stressed the importance of effective communication throughout the incidents. They reported that communication among response agencies was generally effective, but they had difficulty reaching clinicians to provide them with needed guidance. Local and state public health officials were concerned that the capacity of their workforce and clinical laboratories was strained and said that their responses would have been difficult to sustain if the incidents had been more extensive.

The experience of responding to the anthrax incidents also showed aspects of federal preparedness that could be improved. CDC was challenged to both meet heavy resource demands from local and state officials and coordinate the federal public health response in the face of rapidly unfolding anthrax incidents. CDC has acknowledged that although it was effective in its more traditional capacity of supporting local response efforts, it was not fully prepared to manage the federal public health response. CDC served as the focal point for

[5] For information on aspects of the response to the anthrax incidents that are outside the scope of this report, see our reports on those topics: U.S. General Accounting Office, *U.S. Postal Service: Better Guidance Is Needed to Improve Communication Should Anthrax Contamination Occur in the Future*, GAO-03-316 (Washington, D.C.: Apr. 7, 2003); U.S. General Accounting Office, *Capitol Hill Anthrax Incident: EPA's Cleanup Was Successful; Opportunities Exist to Enhance Contract Oversight*, GAO-03-686 (Washington, D.C.: June 4, 2003); and U.S. General Accounting Office, *U.S. Postal Service: Issues Associated with Anthrax Testing at the Wallingford Facility*, GAO-03-787T (Washington, D.C.: May 19, 2003). For a list of our other work related to bioterrorism preparedness, see the list of related products at the end of this report.

communicating critical information during the response to the anthrax incidents and experienced difficulty in managing the voluminous amount of information coming into the agency and in communicating with public health officials, the media, and the public. In addition to straining CDC's resources, the anthrax incidents highlighted both shortcomings in the clinical tools available for responding to anthrax, such as vaccines and drugs, and a lack of training for clinicians on how to recognize and respond to anthrax.

CDC has reviewed its performance during the anthrax incidents, identified areas for improvement, and taken steps to implement those improvements. These include restructuring the Office of the Director, building and staffing an emergency operations center, enhancing the agency's communication infrastructure, and developing and maintaining databases of information on and expertise in biological agents considered most likely to be used in a terrorist attack. CDC has also increased its collaborative efforts with others within and outside of HHS, for example, by creating a permanent position of CDC liaison to the Federal Bureau of Investigation (FBI). CDC has also been working with other federal agencies as well as private organizations to support the development of better clinical tools, including new vaccines and treatments for anthrax and other potential agents of bioterrorism, and increased training for medical care professionals.

Background

Anthrax

Anthrax is an acute infectious disease caused by the spore-forming bacterium called *Bacillus anthracis*. The bacterium is commonly found in the soil, and its spores can remain dormant for many years. Although anthrax can infect humans, it occurs most commonly in plant-eating animals. Human anthrax infections have usually resulted from occupational exposure to infected animals or contaminated animal products, such as wool, hides, or hair. Both human and animal anthrax infections are rare in the United States.

Anthrax infection can take one of three forms: cutaneous, usually through a cut or an abrasion; gastrointestinal, usually by ingesting undercooked contaminated meat; or inhalational, by breathing airborne anthrax spores into the lungs. After the spores enter the body through any of these routes, they germinate into bacteria, which then multiply and secrete toxins that can produce local swelling and tissue death. The symptoms are different for each form and usually occur within 7 days of exposure. Depending on the extent of exposure and its form, a person can be exposed to *Bacillus anthracis* without developing an infection. There are several methods for detecting anthrax spores or the disease itself, for example, nasal swabs for exposure to spores, blood tests for infections, and wet swabs for environmental contamination. CDC does not recommend the use of the nasal swab test to determine whether an individual should be treated, primarily because a negative result (no spores detected) does not exclude the possibility of exposure. Confirmation of anthrax infection or the presence of anthrax spores can require more than one type of test. The disease can be treated with a variety of antimicrobial medications and is not contagious.[6] With proper treatment, fatalities are rare for cutaneous anthrax. For gastrointestinal anthrax, between 25

[6] An antimicrobial medication either kills or slows the growth of microbes.

and 60 percent of cases have resulted in death. For inhalational anthrax, the fatality rate before the 2001 incidents had been approximately 75 percent, even with appropriate antimicrobial medications. An anthrax vaccine is available, but it is indicated for use in individuals at high risk of exposure to anthrax spores, such as laboratory personnel who work with *Bacillus anthracis*.

Because so few instances of inhalational anthrax have occurred, scientific understanding about the number of spores needed to cause infection is still evolving. Before the 2001 incidents, it was estimated that a person would need to inhale thousands of spores to develop an infection. However, based on some of the cases that occurred during the anthrax incidents, experts now believe that the number of spores needed to cause inhalational anthrax could be fewer than that, depending on a person's health and the nature of the spores.

Public Health Response to a Bioterrorist Attack

In the existing model for response to a public health emergency of any type, including a bioterrorist attack, the initial response is generally a local responsibility. This local response can involve multiple jurisdictions in a region, with states providing additional support as needed. Having the necessary resources immediately available at the local level to respond to an emergency can minimize the magnitude of the event and the cost of remediation. In the case of a covert release of a biological agent such as anthrax, it can be days before exposed people start exhibiting signs and symptoms of the disease. The model anticipates that exposed individuals would seek out local clinicians, such as private physicians or medical staff in hospital emergency departments or public clinics. Clinicians would report any illness patterns or diagnostic clues that might indicate an unusual infectious disease outbreak to their state or local health departments. Local and state health departments would collect and monitor data, such as reports from clinicians, for disease trends and evidence of an outbreak. Environmental and clinical samples would be collected for laboratorians[7] to test for possible exposures and identification of illnesses. Epidemiologists[8] in the health departments would use the disease surveillance systems[9] to provide for the ongoing collection, analysis, and dissemination of data to identify unusual patterns of disease. Public health officials would provide needed information to the clinical community, other responders, and the public and would implement control measures to prevent additional cases from occurring. The federal government can also become involved, as requested, by providing assistance with testing of samples and epidemiologic investigations, providing advice on treatment protocols and other technical information, and coordinating a national response.

[7] A laboratorian is one who works in a laboratory; in the medical and allied health professions, a laboratorian examines or performs tests (or supervises such procedures) with various types of chemical and biologic materials, chiefly to aid in the diagnosis, treatment, and control of disease, or as a basis for health and sanitation practices.

[8] An epidemiologist is a specialist in the study of how disease is distributed in populations and the factors that influence or determine this distribution.

[9] Disease surveillance systems provide for the ongoing collection, analysis, and dissemination of health-related data to identify, prevent, and control disease.

CDC's Bioterrorism Response Planning Efforts

As early as 1998, CDC had begun its planning efforts to enhance its capacity to respond effectively to bioterrorism. CDC said it was responsible for providing national leadership in the public health and medical communities in a concerted effort to detect, diagnose, respond to, and prevent illnesses that occur as a result of bioterrorism. In its strategic preparedness and response plan, CDC anticipated that it would need to collaborate with local and state public health partners and other federal agencies in order to strengthen components of the public health infrastructure.[10] As part of this collaboration, CDC initiated a cooperative agreement program in 1999 to enhance state and local bioterrorism preparedness. CDC's planning efforts identified the importance of coordination with the Department of Justice, including the FBI and the National Domestic Preparedness Office. In addition, CDC said that there was ongoing coordination with the Office of Emergency Preparedness within HHS, FDA, NIH, DOD, the Federal Emergency Management Agency (FEMA), and many other partners, including academic institutions and professional organizations. At the time of the anthrax incidents, some of these collaborative efforts were in the planning stage, some were in the form of working groups, and others were limited in scope to areas such as laboratory preparedness, training, or new vaccine research.

CDC was also working to make improvements in various aspects of preparedness and prevention, detection and surveillance, and communication and coordination. At the time of the anthrax incidents, CDC was working on creating diagnostic and epidemiologic performance standards for local and state health departments. In collaboration with NIH and DOD, CDC was encouraging research for the development of new vaccines, antitoxins, and innovative drugs. In addition, CDC had developed a repository of pharmaceuticals and other supplies through the Strategic National Stockpile.[11] CDC was developing educational materials and providing terrorism-related training to epidemiologists, laboratory workers, emergency responders, emergency department personnel, and other front-line health care providers and health and safety personnel.

Through cooperative agreements, CDC was also working to upgrade the surveillance systems of the local and state health departments and investing in the Health Alert Network (HAN)[12] and Epidemic Information Exchange (Epi-X)[13] communication systems.

---

[10] Public health infrastructure is the foundation that supports the planning, delivery, and evaluation of public health activities and is composed of a well-trained public health workforce, effective program and policy evaluation, sufficient epidemiology and surveillance capability to detect outbreaks and monitor incidence of diseases, appropriate response capacity for public health emergencies, effective laboratories, secure information systems, and advanced communication systems.

[11] At the time of the anthrax incidents, the Strategic National Stockpile was known as the National Pharmaceutical Stockpile.

[12] HAN is a nationwide program designed to ensure communication capacity at all local and state health departments (including full Internet connectivity and training), ensure capacity to receive distance learning offerings from CDC and others, and ensure capacity to broadcast and receive health alerts at every level.

[13] Epi-X is a secure, Web-based communication system to enhance bioterrorism preparedness efforts by facilitating the sharing of preliminary information about disease outbreaks and other health events among public health officials across jurisdictions and provide experience in the use of secure communications.

Fall 2001 Anthrax Incidents

In October 2001, an employee of American Media Inc. (AMI) in Florida was diagnosed with inhalational anthrax, the first case in the United States in over two decades. By the end of November 2001, 21 more people had contracted the disease, and 5 people, including the original victim, had died as a result. Although the FBI confirmed the existence of only four letters containing anthrax spores, by December 2001 the Environmental Protection Agency (EPA) had confirmed that over 60 sites, about one third of which were U.S. postal facilities, had been contaminated with anthrax spores.

The cases of inhalational anthrax in Florida, the first epicenter, were thought to have resulted from proximity to opened letters containing anthrax spores, which were never found. (See table 1.) The initial cases of anthrax detected in New York, the second epicenter, were all cutaneous and were also thought to have been associated with opened anthrax letters. The cases detected initially in New Jersey, the third epicenter, were cutaneous and were in postal workers who presumably had not been exposed to opened anthrax letters. Unlike the incidents at other epicenters, which began when cases of anthrax were detected, the incident on Capitol Hill, the fourth epicenter, began with the opening of a letter containing anthrax spores and resulting exposure. The discovery of inhalational anthrax in a postal worker in the Washington, D.C., regional area, the fifth epicenter, revealed that even individuals who had been exposed only to sealed anthrax letters could contract the inhalational form of the disease. Subsequent inhalational cases in Washington, D.C., New Jersey, New York, and Connecticut, the sixth epicenter, underscored that finding. (For a list of key events in the history of the anthrax incidents and the public health response to the incidents, see app. I.)

Table 1: People with Anthrax Infections, Letters Containing Anthrax Spores, and Facilities Contaminated with Anthrax Spores in the Six Epicenters

	Number of infected people		Letter recovered within epicenter	Contaminated facilities
	Cutaneous anthrax	Inhalational anthrax		
Epicenters				
Florida	0	2	No	Yes
New York	7	1	Yes	Yes
New Jersey	4	2	No[a]	Yes
Capitol Hill	0	0	Yes	Yes
Washington, D.C., regional area	0	5	No[a]	Yes
Connecticut	0	1	No	Yes

Source: CDC.

[a] Although no letters were recovered within the New Jersey and Washington, D.C., epicenters themselves, the letters found in the New York and Capitol Hill epicenters have been determined to be the source of the contamination in New Jersey and Washington, D.C.

Although the anthrax incidents were limited to six epicenters on the East Coast, the incidents had national implications. Because mail processed at contaminated postal facilities could be cross-contaminated and end up anywhere in the country, the localized incidents generated concern about white powders found in locations beyond the epicenters and created a demand throughout the nation for public health resources at the local, state, and federal levels.

Local and State Public Health Officials Identified Strengths in Their Responses as Well as Areas for Improvement

Local and state public health officials across the epicenters emphasized the benefits of their planning efforts for promoting a rapid and coordinated response, stressed the importance of effective communication throughout the incidents, and reported that their response capacity was strained and the response would have been difficult to sustain if the incidents had been more extensive.

Local and State Public Health Officials Relied on Plans for Coordinating with a Wide Range of Entities and Identified Areas for Improvement

Local and state public health officials were challenged to coordinate their responses to the anthrax incidents across a wide range of public and private entities, often across more than one local jurisdiction. Officials reported that anticipating local needs in emergency response plans, making those plans operational with formal contracts and agreements, and having experience with other public emergencies or large events improved their ability to mount a rapid and coordinated response. When pieces of this planning process were missing, had not been operationalized, or had not been tested by experience, coordination of the local response was often more difficult.

Epicenters Had Engaged in Some Response Planning but Had Not Anticipated the Full Extent of Coordination That Would Be Needed

Local and state public health officials reported that they had typically planned for coordination of their emergency response but had not fully anticipated the extent to which they would have to coordinate with a wide range of both public and private entities involved in the response to the anthrax incidents, both locally and in other jurisdictions. Among others, public health departments had to coordinate their responses with those of local and federal law enforcement, emergency responders, the postal community, environmental agencies, and clinicians.

Most response plans anticipated the need for public health officials to coordinate with law enforcement and emergency response officials, both within their community and across jurisdictions. In one epicenter, for example, a regional organization of local governments had developed planning guidance that outlined collaborative networks between the public health and emergency response communities needed to strengthen the region's response to an event such as the anthrax incidents.

In contrast, the need to link the public health response with the responses of other public entities affected by the anthrax incidents, such as environmental agencies, military response teams, and the U.S. Postal Service, was less likely to have been anticipated in local response plans. During the response, standard practices for clinical and environmental testing and use of proper protective clothing and equipment needed to be coordinated among public health officials, postal officials, police, firefighters, environmental specialists, and teams from DOD. However, officials reported that in some cases personnel from environmental and military groups were meeting with public health officials for the first time as the response unfolded. When the need for consistency in testing procedures and standards for protective clothing and equipment had not been anticipated, officials sometimes had difficulty agreeing on which procedures and standards to follow. In addition, some plans had not anticipated the need to forge quick relationships between public health departments and local groups affected by the incidents but not expressly mentioned in the plans. During the anthrax incidents, the absence of such a measure proved to be a particular problem for postal officials and postal union representatives. In part due to this absence of proactive plans, coordination between public health and postal officials on many of the details of the response was problematic, and there were difficulties communicating critical information, such as decisions on how and when to provide prophylactic, or preventive, treatment to postal workers.

The need for coordination between public health and private groups affected by the emergency—such as the hospital community—was also not always fully anticipated in local response plans. Public health officials in several areas had to work with local hospitals and other facilities to set up screening and postexposure prophylaxis clinics rapidly, sometimes in less than 24 hours. In this time they had to identify an appropriate site location, design patient flow plans, outline staff needs and responsibilities (medical, pharmacy, counseling, administrative, and facilities operation components), and obtain medications (including dealing with the logistics of breaking down and repackaging bulk medications). Few locations had formally addressed all of these issues before the anthrax incidents, but those that had addressed at least some of them reported being able to respond more rapidly.

Some Aspects of Response Plans Had Been Made Operational and Increased Officials' Ability to Coordinate a Rapid Response

Officials relied on a variety of formal agreements, such as memoranda of understanding and legal contracts, to address the needs identified in their planning documents. These needs included coordination across disciplines and jurisdictions, access to scientific information, and human resources support. Local officials reported that putting agreements and contracts into place to address these needs strengthened their preparedness both by solidifying links with their public and private partners and by helping them identify weaknesses that could be addressed prior to an emergency. When systems had not been put into place to support plans, coordination of response efforts was more difficult.

Formal agreements had often been put into place to support coordination among officials within communities and across jurisdictions, but some aspects of plans that were important for coordinating the response had not yet been made operational. For example, one official reported having arranged to link surveillance and environmental health personnel with law enforcement officials during criminal investigations in the event of an anthrax attack. Another official had already established agreements with local counterparts to provide access to prophylaxis. Officials reported that when formal contacts between officials had not been established, coordination with counterparts in their community and other jurisdictions during the incidents often relied on personal relationships.

While some public health departments reported having systems in place to ensure ready access to the scientific information needed to make decisions and provide information to the media and the public, many reported that they did not. Officials reported that planning ahead and then taking the necessary steps to compile available scientific information—including what was known about anthrax, procedures for testing exposure to anthrax, treatment protocols, and standards for the types of protective clothing and equipment that are appropriate for first responders—were important for responding rapidly and reducing confusion across the parties involved in the response.

Officials stated that during the response they relied on existing mutual aid agreements or contracts that gave them access to staff for screening and mass care clinics, allowed the state to pull local epidemiologists to support the state response, and addressed licensure issues for staff brought in from other states. However, these agreements were not always in place, or only partially covered the needs of the situation, and some officials had to spend time dealing with issues that could have been addressed before the event. For example, an official in one epicenter reported that because a state of emergency had not been declared in the jurisdiction, there was no system to pay for food for staff who were working 24-hour shifts in prophylaxis clinics. Several officials in other localities reported that systems had not been put into place to authorize payment for overtime work in both public health departments and laboratories. In addition, one health department received offers of volunteer help from many physicians, pharmacists, nurses, epidemiologists, and other concerned citizens. However, it could not use the volunteers because it did not have a volunteer management system to train providers and verify credentials.

Experience with Drills and Responding to Emergencies Allowed Officials to Identify Areas for Improvement in Their Plans

Experience with drills and responding to public health emergencies helped officials identify weaknesses in their plans. These officials stated that drills ranging from tabletop to full-scale exercises were useful for testing coordination and response capacities both locally and regionally. Public health officials also reported that their experience in dealing with hoax letters and false alarms proved useful, particularly in supporting coordination with the law enforcement community. In major metropolitan areas, experience with large events, such as political conventions, forced local public health departments to develop their emergency response plans and put the necessary agreements in place to support those plans. Experience with public health emergencies—including natural disasters and outbreaks of infectious disease such as West Nile virus—also allowed officials to work on coordinating their responses across multiple sites, test their surveillance systems, and establish links with other public and private entities.

Where previous experience had not allowed officials to identify and address shortcomings of their plans, the anthrax incidents tended to uncover weaknesses. For example, one local public health official reported that although the agency had planned how to set up a prophylaxis clinic it had not actually exercised getting people through the testing and prophylaxis process. During the anthrax response, it took significantly longer than the agency had anticipated to obtain test results from overwhelmed laboratories. This official said that if the agency had known how long it was going to take to get laboratory results, it would have provided the first doses of prophylaxis for a longer duration to take into account the additional time required to obtain test results. Another official reported that the agency's experience with setting up a prophylaxis clinic during the anthrax response taught the agency how to select more appropriate sites for mass vaccination or prophylaxis clinics in emergency situations. Experience also revealed shortcomings in regional coordination. Several officials noted that although some plans for coordination across jurisdictions were in place, they had not been exercised, and so the relationships to support coordination had not been formed or tested.

Communicating Effectively during the Incidents Was Challenging

Local officials identified communication among responders and with the public during the anthrax incidents as a challenge, both in terms of having the necessary communication channels and in terms of making the necessary information available for distribution. Good communication can minimize an emergency, improve response, and reassure the public. Officials reported that although communication among local responders was generally effective, there were problems in communicating with some hospitals and physicians. They also reported that dealing with the media and communicating messages to the public were also challenging.

Communication among Response Agencies Was Generally Viewed as Effective

Communication among local and state response agencies was generally perceived to be effective and helped keep agency officials informed and the public health response coordinated. Channels of communication between public health agencies and other responders—including law enforcement and emergency management agencies, hazardous material units, and neighboring state public health agencies—were already in existence at the time of the anthrax incidents. Regular conference calls, which were initiated during the incidents, were used to distribute information, raise issues, and answer questions.

In addition to telephone calls, local and state public health offices relied on fax machines and the Internet to send and receive information during the incidents. Most local health departments, however, noted that they did not have backup communication systems that could be used in case everyday systems became unavailable. In addition, public health workers did not generally have cell phones, pagers, or laptop computers, which could provide the means to keep working if it became necessary to vacate a building during a crisis. In one epicenter, when an agency had to evacuate its quarters during the incidents and workers could not be at their desks, many of its communication systems (in addition to the information stored in the office in electronic formats) became unavailable. Several local agencies that did not have backup systems available at the time of the anthrax incidents told us they have concluded that it is important to invest in such systems to be prepared for any future public health emergencies.

Local response agencies generally got the information they requested from other local agencies. For example, in one epicenter, police and fire departments were given specific protocols for handling suspicious samples and triaging them for the laboratory. However, there were instances in which they did not get needed information. For example, a local emergency response official stated that the local fire department did not know what protective equipment (such as masks and gloves) firefighters should wear when responding to a suspected anthrax incident. The fire department turned to the local health department for answers, but the health department took weeks to release the protocol.

Flow of Information to Clinicians Was Problematic

State and local officials reported difficulty providing needed information to some hospitals and physicians in a timely way, and members of the medical community expressed concern about the timeliness of the information they received. Physicians recognized that they lacked experience with anthrax and were particularly concerned about missing a diagnosis because of its high fatality rate. They expected to be given rapid and specific instructions from public health officials about how to recognize and treat people who had been exposed. They wanted guidelines, for example, on how to diagnose inhalational anthrax and how to advise individuals who worked in post offices. Hospitals in one epicenter reported receiving daily influxes of people with flulike symptoms. Because these hospitals were seeking guidance on how to distinguish between influenza and anthrax symptoms, the hospital association in the area initiated daily conference calls with concerned clinicians. The purpose of these calls was to collect questions to ask other organizations, such as CDC, to coordinate consistent answers to questions from the public, and to share information about clinical approaches.

Some of the ways in which local public health agencies tried to communicate with hospitals and physicians were regarded as relatively effective by the agencies, but no method worked well for all targeted recipients. Health departments used various means to make relevant materials available to hospitals and physicians, including sending faxes or e-mail messages, posting relevant information on their Web sites, distributing CD-ROMs, and setting up hotlines. In one state, which had no confirmed anthrax infections but numerous false alarms, the state public health department faxed critical information to hospitals throughout the state. Officials in the department reported that while this system was useful in disseminating information it was insufficient because it did not provide a means of receiving information from the hospitals. E-mail worked well for institutions, but it was an ineffective way of communicating with physicians, especially those who did not have a hospital-based practice. Several local public health officials told us that many private physicians did not have e-mail or Web access. Because electronic messages were not a feasible way of communicating with many clinicians, there was no way to get timely information about anthrax to them. Some primary care physicians were difficult to reach by any mass communication method or even individually because public health officials sometimes did not have up-to-date rosters of their telephone numbers. Officials in one state said they realized during the incidents that they did not have a way to send information directly to dermatologists, a group of specialists who were especially important for detecting the cutaneous form of anthrax infection. Because localities were unable to reach all physicians directly, government agencies relied on physicians and associations who did receive the information to serve as conduits. However, government and association officials agreed that this method did not provide complete coverage of all physicians.

Criminal Investigation Sometimes Hindered Flow of Information to Officials and the Public

Local officials reported that the criminal investigation of the anthrax incidents sometimes hindered their ability to obtain information they needed to conduct their public health response. For example, public health officials in one epicenter said that they were unable to get certain information from the FBI because the local public health officials lacked security clearances. They said that if they had received more detailed information earlier about the nature of the anthrax spores in the envelopes, it might have affected how their agencies were responding. In addition, a laboratory director in one of the epicenters reported that the criminal investigation led to constraints on his ability to communicate laboratory results to clinicians.

Just as information was not provided to government agencies because of law enforcement considerations, officials stated that criminal aspects of the incidents complicated the distribution of information to the public. Officials expressed concern about the necessity of withholding some information from the public. One official reported that communication with the public was constrained when the situation became a criminal investigation. She was concerned that information the public needed to understand its risk was no longer being provided. Officials in one epicenter told us that they were concerned that constraints on the ability of local public health departments to communicate could lead to a loss of credibility. More generally, officials reported that fear in the community could have been reduced if they had been able to release more information to the media and the public.

Supplying Information to Meet Needs of Media and Local Public Was Challenging

Local and state officials reported that although they were generally successful in persuading people to seek treatment, they encountered difficulties in providing needed information to the media and local public during the anthrax incidents. Because the incidents were taking place in many locations, local communications were complicated by the public's exposure to information about other localities and from the national media.

Local and state officials realized that they needed to use the media to disseminate information to the public and that they needed to be responsive to the media so that the information the media were providing was accurate. Public health and other government officials in the epicenters held regular press conferences to keep the public informed about local developments, made officials available to respond to media requests, and developed informational materials so that the media and the public could be better informed. Several officials stated that the media helped in publicizing sources of information such as hotlines and specific information such as details about who should seek treatment and where to go for it. However, media analysts have also noted that the media were sometimes responsible for providing incorrect information. For example, one official said that when the media reported that nasal swabbing was the test for anthrax, individuals sought unnecessary nasal swab testing from emergency rooms, physicians, and the health department, and thereby diverted medical and laboratory resources from medical care that was required elsewhere.

Communication with the public was further complicated by the evolving nature of the incidents and the local public's exposure to information from other localities and the national media. Comparisons of actions taken by officials at different points in time and in different areas caused the public to question the consistency and fairness of actions taken in their locale. For example, the affected public in some epicenters wondered why they were being given doxycycline for prophylaxis instead of ciprofloxacin, which had been heralded in the media as the drug of choice for the prevention of inhalational anthrax and used earlier in other epicenters. CDC's initial recommendation for ciprofloxacin was made because ciprofloxacin was judged to be most likely to be effective against any naturally occurring strain of anthrax and had already been approved by FDA for use in postexposure prophylaxis for inhalational anthrax. However, when it was determined that doxycycline was equally effective against the strain of anthrax in the letters and following FDA's announcement that doxycycline was approved for inhalational anthrax, the recommendation was changed. This change was made because of doxycycline's lower risk for side effects and lower cost and because of concerns that strains of bacteria resistant to ciprofloxacin could emerge if tens of thousands of people were taking it. In epicenters where prophylaxis was initiated after the recommendation had changed, officials followed the new recommendation and gave doxycycline to affected people. Local officials were challenged to explain the switch and address concerns raised by affected groups about apparently differential treatment. One local official described the importance of explaining that the switch was also taking place even in locations that had started with ciprofloxacin.

Response Capacity Was Strained and Would Have Been Difficult to Sustain

Elements of the local and state public health response systems—including the public health department and laboratory workforce as well as laboratories—were strained by the anthrax incidents to an extent that many local and state officials told us that they might not have been able to manage if the crisis had lasted longer. The anthrax incidents required extended hours for many public health workers investigating the incidents, as well as the assignment of new tasks, including the staffing of hotlines, to some workers. Aside from problems of workforce capacity, some clinical laboratories were not prepared in terms of equipment, supplies, or available laboratory protocols to test for anthrax, and most of them were unprepared for and overwhelmed by the large number of environmental samples they received for testing. The systems experienced these stresses in spite of assistance from CDC and DOD, and temporary transfers of local, and in some cases regional, resources.

Public Health Workers Were Overwhelmed with Work

During the anthrax incidents, the workload increased greatly at local and state health departments and laboratories and across the country. The departments heightened their disease surveillance, investigated false alarms and hoaxes as well as potential threats, tested large numbers of samples, and performed other duties such as answering calls on telephone hotlines that were set up to respond to questions from the public. Health departments across the nation received thousands of such calls. For example, officials at one location told us that they received 25,000 calls over a 2-week period during the crisis. Nine states—Colorado, Connecticut, Louisiana, Maryland, Montana, North Dakota, Tennessee, Wisconsin, and Wyoming—reported to CDC that during the week of October 21 to 27, 2001, they received a total of 2,817 bioterrorism-related calls. These nine states also reported that during that week they conducted approximately 25 investigations per state and had from 8 to 30 state personnel engaged full-time in the responses in each state.

Some local and state health departments had to borrow workers from other parts of their agencies or from outside of their agencies, such as from CDC and DOD, to meet the greater demands for surveillance, investigation, laboratory testing, and other duties related to the incidents. Several agencies realized that they lacked staff in particular specialties, such as environmental epidemiology. Some state public health departments did not have enough epidemiologists to investigate the suspected cases in their localities and had to borrow staff from other programs. Health workers were pulled from other jobs to work in the field or to staff the telephone hotlines. Staff borrowed from other parts of the agency were sometimes unable to fulfill their traditional public health duties, such as working on prevention of sexually transmitted diseases, and some routine work was delayed. In spite of the borrowing, staff at some agencies worked long hours over a number of weeks. In some cases, state laboratories had to borrow staff from various parts of their health department because laboratory workers were overwhelmed and the laboratories required staffing for 24 hours a day, 7 days a week. In some locations, CDC provided epidemiologists and laboratorians to help fill gaps in staff.

Some borrowed workers had to be trained for their new duties while the incidents were ongoing. Some workers had to be trained or cross-trained in two fields, requiring additional time from other staff and resources from the department. Some borrowed staff had to be trained for the specific tasks required by the incidents. Finding sufficient numbers of people who were appropriately trained or could be efficiently trained to staff the telephone hotlines effectively was also a challenge. Local officials reported that even if sufficient staff were found, calls were not always handled effectively, especially when the caller needed mental health services.

Many officials we interviewed were concerned about their ability to deal with demand on staff in future crises. Since the anthrax incidents, some states have sent members of their staff for additional training. Some officials emphasized that surge capacity should be flexible to ensure preparedness for various types of future bioterrorism incidents.

Laboratories Handled Huge Volumes of Samples, and Some Were Underequipped to Do So

In addition to overwhelming the laboratory workforce, the large influx of samples strained the physical capacity of the laboratories. Public health laboratories around the country tested thousands of white powders and other environmental samples as well as clinical samples. According to CDC, during the anthrax incidents, laboratories within the Laboratory Response Network[14] tested more than 120,000 samples, the bulk of which were environmental samples. Officials from one state told us that its laboratories did not have the capacity to handle the volume of work they received. Some local and state public health laboratories could not analyze anthrax samples because of limitations of equipment, supplies, or laboratory protocols. For example, in some states there were a limited number of biological safety cabinets, which were needed to prevent inhalation of anthrax spores by laboratory workers during the testing of samples. Some laboratories did not have the chemicals needed to conduct the appropriate tests. In some states, none of the state laboratories could conduct an essential diagnostic test for anthrax, the polymerase chain reaction test. In another state, only one of three state laboratories could perform this test. Some state and local laboratories were not prepared to take the safety precautions required to test samples for anthrax. Local laboratories were even less capable of doing anthrax testing. Samples for confirmatory testing

[14] The Laboratory Response Network was established in 1999 by CDC, DOD, and the Association of Public Health Laboratories to maintain state-of-the-art capabilities for biological agent identification and characterization. The network is a multilevel system designed to link local and state public health laboratories with advanced capacity clinical, military, veterinary, agricultural, water, and food-testing laboratories. About 100 laboratories participate in the network, with at least one network laboratory in each state.

were sent to CDC or to DOD's USAMRIID. In addition to performing confirmatory testing, DOD also provided other laboratory support to state and local officials. For example, the samples from one epicenter were sent to DOD, and the department sent mobile laboratories to two other epicenters to assist with testing samples.

Moreover, although some laboratories were relatively well prepared to test clinical samples, they were not expecting the hundreds of environmental samples they received and did not have protocols prepared for testing them. It was the volume of these environmental samples, rather than the volume of the clinical samples, that overwhelmed the laboratories. Among the environmental samples, there were white powder samples that arrived without any assessment by law enforcement as to the level of threat they posed. At least one state laboratory developed protocols so that law enforcement personnel could triage samples, thereby increasing the likelihood that only those samples with a relatively high threat level would be forwarded to the laboratory for further testing. Even where protocols for testing these samples were available, it was a time-consuming and unfamiliar task for the laboratory to label them, track their progress, and ensure that their results were reported to the appropriate authority.

Experience Showed Aspects of Federal Preparedness That Could Be Improved

CDC led the federal public health response to the anthrax incidents, and the experience showed aspects of federal preparedness that could be improved. During the anthrax incidents, CDC was designated to act on behalf of HHS in providing national leadership in the public health and medical communities. As the lead agency in the federal public health response, CDC had to not only provide public health expertise but also manage the public health response efforts across epicenters and among other federal agencies. While local and state officials reported that CDC's support of their responses to the rapidly unfolding anthrax incidents at the local and state levels was generally effective, CDC acknowledged that it was not fully prepared for the challenge of coordinating the public health response across the federal agencies. CDC experienced difficulty serving as the focal point for communicating critical information during the response. In addition to straining CDC's resources, the anthrax incidents highlighted shortcomings in the clinical tools available for responding to anthrax, such as vaccines and drugs, and a lack of training for clinicians on how to recognize and respond to anthrax.

CDC Provided Support to Meet Heavy Resource Demands from Local and State Officials

CDC effectively responded to heavy resource demands from state and local officials to support the local responses. CDC reported that its support activities included surveillance; clinical, epidemiologic, and environmental investigation; laboratory work; communications; coordination with law enforcement; medical management; administration of prophylaxis; monitoring of adverse events; and decontamination. As new epicenters became involved, CDC dispersed additional agency staff to assist local and state health departments and other groups playing a role in the response efforts, eventually deploying more than 350 employees to the six epicenters. In addition, because even the perception of danger required a public health response, CDC also provided assistance as requested in localities beyond the epicenters. From October 8 to 31, 2001, CDC's emergency response center received 8,860 telephone inquiries from all 50 states, the District of Columbia, Puerto Rico, Guam, and 22 foreign countries. CDC's callers included health care workers, local and state health departments, the public, and police, fire, and emergency departments and included requests for information about anthrax vaccines, bioterrorism prevention, and the use of personal protective equipment. Thus CDC not only provided resources to the epicenters but also had to coordinate local efforts nationwide.

Local public health offices required varying levels of assistance from CDC. For example, in one epicenter local officials looked to CDC to lead the epidemiologic investigation and relied primarily on CDC staff. In contrast, local officials in another epicenter led the local disease outbreak investigation and control effort and CDC staff supplemented a large local team. In most of the epicenters, the team sent by CDC included Epidemic Intelligence Service (EIS) officers, who are specially trained epidemiologists, to help with the investigation. The team's epidemiologic investigation used the traditional two-pronged approach in which it completely investigated either the case or the circumstance of a confirmed exposure and conducted intensive surveillance to identify any other anthrax cases or exposures. Laboratory testing proved to be an important tool in the epidemiologic investigation, and the CDC team also included laboratorians, who assisted with laboratory testing. In one epicenter, CDC also sent one of its anthrax experts to provide guidance and assist the local and state officials.

CDC Reported It Was Not Fully Prepared to Coordinate the Federal Public Health Response

In addition to playing its traditional role of supporting local and state public health departments, CDC also was confronted with the challenge of coordinating the public health activities of multiple federal agencies involved in the response, a task for which it acknowledged it was not wholly prepared. CDC described having to create an ad hoc emergency response center in an auditorium from which to manage the federal public health response, which involved numerous agencies. These included FDA, which, among other activities, provided guidance on treatment and addressed drug and blood safety issues. In addition, NIH provided scientific expertise on anthrax. CDC also coordinated with federal agencies working on the environmental and law enforcement aspects of the response efforts. DOD was responsible for testing all of the anthrax letters that were recovered and was involved in the transportation and testing of environmental samples as well as the cleanup of contaminated buildings. EPA was in charge of the cleanup of contaminated sites. FEMA assisted the President's Office of Homeland Security in establishing and supporting an emergency support team. The FBI led the criminal investigation.

Although CDC's planning efforts prior to the anthrax incidents had identified the importance of coordination with other federal agencies for an effective response to bioterrorism, and CDC had developed some working groups among federal agencies, CDC sometimes had to adjust its response as events unfolded to facilitate coordination of more practical issues such as conducting simultaneous investigations in the field. For example,

CDC told us that in one epicenter both CDC and the FBI, which needed to collect samples for the forensic investigation, identified the need to gain a better understanding of one another's work. During the incidents, CDC provided a liaison to the FBI, and the agencies worked together to collect laboratory samples. Since the anthrax incidents, CDC has held joint training with the FBI to discuss what they learned from their experience that could facilitate working together in the future.

CDC has made several efforts to improve coordination since the anthrax incidents, including major structural changes within the agency, creation of a permanent emergency operations center (EOC), and increased collaborative efforts with others within and outside of HHS. Officials point to the creation of the Office of Terrorism Preparedness and Emergency Response, which is part of the Office of the Director, as a major change. The primary services of this office are to provide strategic direction for CDC to support terrorism preparedness and response efforts, secure and position resources to support activities, and ensure that systems are in place to monitor performance and manage accountability. The office manages the cooperative agreement program to enhance local and state preparedness and jointly manages the Strategic National Stockpile with the Department of Homeland Security. The office also manages the EOC, which was created to promote quicker and better-coordinated responses to public health emergencies across the country and around the globe. The EOC is staffed 24 hours a day, 7 days a week, and the staff includes officials from FEMA, DOD, and other agencies. CDC also created a permanent position of CDC liaison to the FBI to increase collaboration with that agency.

CDC Experienced Difficulty Serving as Focal Point for Communicating Critical Information during Response to Anthrax Incidents

CDC served as the focal point for information flow during the anthrax incidents, but experienced some difficulty in fulfilling that role. In addition to the varied responsibilities involved in leading the public health response, the agency concurrently had to collect and analyze the large amount of incoming information on the anthrax incidents, assemble and analyze the available scientific information on anthrax, and produce guidance and other information based on its analyses for dissemination to officials, other responders, the media, and the public. CDC officials reported that the agency had difficulty producing and disseminating this guidance rapidly as well as difficulty conveying information to the media and the public.

CDC Had Difficulty Managing the Influx of Information to Produce and Disseminate Guidance Rapidly

CDC officials acknowledged that the agency was not always able to produce guidance as quickly as it would have liked. When the incidents began, it did not have a nationwide list of outside experts on anthrax, and it had not compiled all of the relevant scientific literature on anthrax. Consequently, CDC had to do time-consuming research to gather background information to inform its decisions, which slowed the development of its guidance. CDC has since compiled background information and lists of experts not only for anthrax but also for the other biological agents identified as having the greatest potential for adverse public health impact with mass casualties in a terrorist attack, and it has made the background information available on its Web site.[15]

CDC officials reported that CDC also had difficulty compiling the information it received during the incidents. Although CDC's role as focal point for information was a familiar one, the magnitude of information it received was unusual. CDC received a tremendous amount of information via e-mail, phone, fax, and news media reports from such sources as the agencies and organizations in the epicenters of the incidents, public health departments not in the epicenters, other federal agencies, and international public health organizations. CDC also received information from its staff in the field, but encountered some problems in those communications. Agency officials have said there were communication problems between epidemiologic staff in the field and at headquarters, which CDC attempted to address by holding "mission briefings" through its emergency response center; however, these briefings were not conducted regularly. CDC's efforts to manage all of this incoming information and associated internal communication problems were complicated by its concurrent responsibility for coordinating the day-to-day activities involved in the federal public health response to the unfolding incidents.

According to CDC, both clinical and environmental guidance was developed during the incidents by using working groups of six to eight employees who were subject matter experts. Keeping up with the influx of new information that was being acquired daily proved to be a challenge for these working groups. CDC officials told us that no group at CDC was responsible for collecting and analyzing all of the data that were coming in and that few people at CDC had time to read their e-mail messages during the incidents. Since the incidents, CDC has established teams of scientists from inside and outside CDC whose only role is to review and analyze information during a crisis; CDC does not intend for these teams to be involved in day-to-day response operations.

As the working groups incorporated new information into their analyses, the guidance they were producing changed accordingly. For example, as the epidemiologic investigation expanded, CDC had to revise its assessment of the risk of developing inhalational anthrax from letters containing anthrax spores. Early on, CDC was acting on the theory that there was little risk of contracting inhalational anthrax from sealed letters. The incidents in the Washington, D.C., regional area, the fifth epicenter, represented a turning point in the epidemiologic investigation. The discovery of inhalational anthrax in a postal worker who presumably had been in contact only with sealed anthrax letters required CDC to revise its assessment. From this point on, CDC presumed that any exposure would put an individual at risk and changed its recommendation regarding who should get prophylaxis accordingly. CDC began to recommend prophylaxis for all individuals who had been in contact with sealed as well as unsealed anthrax letters, whereas earlier the agency had not been recommending such treatment unless an individual had been exposed to an opened letter.

Initially, CDC relied on the HAN communication system and its *Morbidity and Mortality Weekly Report* (*MMWR*) publication to disseminate its guidance and other information; however, during the incidents there were difficulties with both of these methods. At the time of the incidents, all state health departments were connected to the HAN system. However, only 13 states were connected to all of their local health jurisdictions, and therefore HAN

[15] These agents, which are labeled Category A agents, are anthrax, botulism, plague, smallpox, tularemia, and viral hemorrhagic fevers.

messages could not reach many local areas. Some states were satisfied with the information they received via HAN, but others claimed they did not get much information from HAN and what they did get was incomplete. During the incidents, CDC expanded its list of HAN recipients to include additional organizations, including medical associations. *MMWR* is issued on a weekly basis, and so the information in the latest issue was not always completely up-to-date for incidents that were unfolding by the hour. For example, information published in *MMWR* on October 26, 2001, contained the notice that the information was current as of October 24, 2001. In addition to these structural barriers to getting information out quickly to those who needed it, CDC's internal process of clearing information before issuance through HAN or *MMWR* was time-consuming. CDC has since changed its clearing process so that information can get out faster. The agency also made a number of other changes during the incidents to address some of the difficulties it encountered in providing information to the public health departments and clinicians. These included bringing in professionals from other communication departments in CDC to help get information out quickly, issuing press releases twice a day, and holding telebriefings. Since the incidents, CDC has taken actions to expand its communication capacity, including developing an emergency communication plan, increasing the number of health experts on staff, and establishing a pressroom, in which the Director of CDC gives press briefings on public health efforts. In addition, it has developed, and posted to its Web site, information to assist local and state health officials in detecting and treating individuals infected with agents considered likely to be used in a bioterrorist attack.

CDC Had Difficulty Conveying Information to Media and Public

During the anthrax incidents, the media and the public looked to CDC as the source for health-related information, but CDC was not always able to successfully convey the information that it had. Media analysts and other commentators have asserted that although CDC officials were the most authoritative spokespersons they were not initially the most visible. In an October 2001 nationwide poll, respondents indicated that they considered the Director of CDC and the U.S. Surgeon General to be better sources of reliable information about the outbreak of disease caused by bioterrorism than other federal officials mentioned in the survey.

Another problem CDC encountered in its efforts to communicate messages to the public was difficulty in conveying the uncertainty associated with the messages, that is, the caveat that although the messages were based on the best available information, they were subject to change when new facts became known. As a bioterrorist event unfolds and new information is learned, recommendations about who is at risk and how people should be treated may change, and the public needs to be prepared that changes may occur. Local officials and academics have criticized CDC's communication of uncertainty during the anthrax incidents. CDC officials have acknowledged that they were unsuccessful in clearly communicating their degree of uncertainty as knowledge was evolving during the incidents. For example, although there were internal disagreements at CDC over the appropriate length of prophylaxis, this uncertainty was not effectively conveyed to the public. Consequently, in December 2001, when many people were finishing the 60-day antimicrobial regimen called for in CDC's guidance, the public questioned CDC's announcement that patients might want to consider an additional 40 days of antimicrobials. Since the incidents, CDC officials have acknowledged the necessity of expressing uncertainty in terms the public can understand and appending appropriate caveats to the agency's statements.

Anthrax Incidents Strained Some Aspects of Federal Response Capacity

The anthrax incidents highlighted some of the strengths of the federal public health response capacity, while also reflecting some of its limitations. CDC's experience with epidemiologic investigations was drawn on extensively and effectively, and the Laboratory Response Network played an important role. Not all the clinical tools that were needed to identify, treat, and prevent anthrax infection were available, and those that were available had shortcomings. Although CDC's bioterrorism preparedness training program for clinicians had begun at the time of the incidents, most clinicians had not yet been trained to recognize and report anthrax infection.

CDC's Epidemiologic and Laboratory Resources Were Strained

CDC's skills in disease investigation were heavily relied on during the anthrax incidents. CDC teams worked with local and state public health departments and law enforcement to determine what happened with each case. CDC's EIS was an important component of the agency's response. The availability of trained epidemiologists enabled CDC to send numbers of them to each epicenter to provide temporary staff to help investigate the nature and extent of the local incident. CDC reported that because of the number of epicenters and calls for assistance from other localities, its staff, both at headquarters and in the field, were spread thin. The level of assistance provided by CDC depended on the needs of the local public health departments and therefore varied considerably by location. For example, while CDC epidemiologists augmented the staff of some local and state health departments who would have been severely overtaxed without CDC's help, the agency characterized its role in one epicenter as supplementary to that epicenter's team of epidemiologists.

The Laboratory Response Network proved to be an asset, and some state and local officials told us they were satisfied with the laboratory response during the anthrax incidents. At that time, CDC laboratories, like many of the laboratories in the network, were inundated with samples and operated 24 hours a day to help epidemiologists determine exposure and risk by testing samples to confirm cases. From October 2001 to December 2001, the network laboratories processed more than 120,000 samples for *Bacillus anthracis*. Public health laboratories other than those at CDC tested 69 percent of these samples, DOD laboratories tested 25 percent, and CDC laboratories tested 6 percent. In addition to testing samples at its laboratories, DOD also assisted the epicenters by providing personnel for laboratories in the epicenters and at CDC and operating portable laboratories to support local investigations. In addition to testing samples, CDC laboratories distributed chemicals needed for testing samples to network laboratories and developed a new testing method that permitted better diagnostics from biopsy samples. CDC used the network to send information to state bioterrorism response coordinators in local and state laboratories. State laboratories also communicated with each other and with CDC by using the network.

However, there were signs of strain in the Laboratory Response Network. USAMRIID officials told us that USAMRIID, as well as other military and civilian laboratories, is set up to process clinical samples and was unprepared to process the volume and types of environmental samples that it received. They noted that many of the procedures for obtaining environmental samples from objects, such as keyboards and telephones, had never been standardized. Officials reported that they spent a great deal of time developing and validating these procedures as the incidents unfolded. In addition, DOD laboratory officials told us that they had to process overflow samples from overwhelmed laboratories at CDC and in the epicenters. DOD officials expressed concern about dependence on DOD laboratory resources for civilian emergencies, noting that in wartime DOD's laboratories are needed to support military operations.

The Strategic National Stockpile was also an asset in CDC's response efforts. The anthrax incidents underscored the benefits of having a system in place to transport antimicrobials and vaccines quickly to areas that need them during emergencies. The Strategic National Stockpile program delivered antimicrobial medications for postexposure prophylaxis and provided for the transportation of anthrax vaccine, clinical and environmental samples, and CDC personnel, including epidemiologists, laboratory scientists, pathologists, and special teams of researchers.

Available Clinical Tools Had Shortcomings

Not all of the clinical tools that physicians needed to identify, treat, and prevent anthrax infection were available, and those that were had shortcomings. Clinicians did not suspect and had difficulty promptly diagnosing anthrax because of their inexperience with the disease and because of the nonspecific nature of its presenting symptoms. Cutaneous anthrax can be confused with cellulitis or a spider bite. Inhalational anthrax is difficult to distinguish from other respiratory illnesses, such as pneumonia or influenza. Routine laboratory and radiological testing did not always clearly signal anthrax infection, and, even after physicians did suspect it, the laboratory tests needed to confirm it were time-consuming, laborious, and required that samples be sent to specialized laboratories. Diagnostic tests that are more accurate and can yield results more quickly are in development.

Treatment for anthrax infection was available, but it was not effective in almost half of the inhalational cases. Both inhalational and cutaneous anthrax, once diagnosed, were treated with a combination of intravenous antimicrobial medications. All of the patients with cutaneous anthrax recovered, but 5 of the 11 patients with inhalational anthrax did not. The drugs worked by killing the bacteria that develop from anthrax spores following germination of those spores in the body. However, anthrax bacteria produce toxins, and no treatments were available that could destroy these toxins. For this reason, the antimicrobial drugs used to treat inhalational anthrax were ineffective in those patients in whom the bacteria had already produced too much toxin by the time treatment was initiated. CDC is working with other agencies within HHS, such as NIH, and other federal agencies, including DOD, to support the development of new treatments for anthrax and other potential agents of bioterrorism.

Methods of prophylaxis for people exposed to anthrax spores were available and apparently effective, but there were several difficulties with these methods. There was uncertainty about how to assess exposure to determine who should be given prophylaxis; initially only one drug had been approved for prophylaxis, and it was approved only for prophylaxis of inhalational anthrax; the optimal length of prophylaxis for those thought to have been exposed to anthrax spores was unknown; prophylactic drugs had to be taken for months and had side effects; and the anthrax vaccine requires more than one dose, had not been approved for postexposure prophylaxis, and was in short supply. Nasal swabs and blood tests were used early in the investigation to assess exposure, but these were not reliable methods. When there was uncertainty about who was exposed or how great their risk from exposure was, prophylaxis was sometimes recommended for all workers in a facility with some contamination, regardless of how close to the contamination the workers had been. This prophylaxis often started with an initial supply of medication while test results were awaited. For example, some people were given a 10-day supply of drugs and asked to return within 10 days to learn whether they needed to continue taking the drugs. Initially, CDC, with advice from NIH, recommended prophylaxis for 60 days.[16] The drugs had side effects, and the rate of compliance with the regimen was typically about 40 percent. Since the incidents, federal agencies have been developing and evaluating tools for detecting anthrax spores. Such tests could enable field workers to make better initial assessments of exposure at particular locations to determine who should get prophylaxis. CDC is working with other federal agencies to support the development of new methods of prophylaxis for anthrax and other potential agents of bioterrorism.

HHS reported that at the time of the anthrax incidents no system or data collection instruments existed for monitoring the nearly 10,000 people who were receiving prophylaxis and thus it did not have a way to collect information on the compliance with, adverse events from, or effectiveness of prophylaxis. CDC attempted to collect this information retrospectively, but acknowledged that this method is not optimal. To improve preparedness for future incidents, CDC and FDA have created a post-event surveillance working group that is responsible for developing a system capable of collecting this kind of data.

Few Clinicians Had Been Trained to Recognize Anthrax

During the anthrax incidents, it became apparent that few clinicians had been trained to recognize anthrax infections. In November 2000, CDC had created a national training plan for bioterrorism preparedness and response. The plan outlined training required to implement the agency's Bioterrorism Event Response Operational Plan and strategies for training public health and medical professionals in collaboration with partners (chiefly public health organizations and professional groups such as the American Medical Association). At the time of the anthrax incidents, CDC had been implementing the plan for less than a year, and relatively few people had been trained: CDC reports that by October 2001 about 12,000 physicians, nurses, and other medical professionals had completed the programs. However, CDC estimated that during the incidents more than one million medical professionals participated in its anthrax-related training programs via satellite, Web, video, and phone. In addition to CDC's training programs, which continue to be available, CDC collaborates with professional organizations, such as the American Medical Association and the American Nurses Association, to provide training for their members, and other federal agencies present training programs on bioterrorism (for example, AHRQ) or fund training programs on bioterrorism (for example, the Health Resources and Services Administration).

---

[16] Later, CDC recommended expanding prophylaxis for those already on it to include an additional 40 days of antimicrobial drugs, with or without three doses of the anthrax vaccine.

Concluding Observations

The anthrax incidents of 2001 required an unprecedented public health response. The specific nature of the incidents and the nature of the response varied across the epicenters and other localities across the country. In each epicenter, local officials had to coordinate responses that were a combination of local, state, and federal efforts. In addition, local public health officials in the epicenters were challenged to mount an intensive response that included identifying and treating people already infected with anthrax as well as people who had been exposed and could become infected, identifying contaminated areas and preventing additional people from being exposed, processing thousands of samples suspected of containing anthrax, and responding to thousands of calls from concerned members of their communities.

The public health response to the anthrax incidents both demonstrated the benefit of public health preparedness measures already in place or under way at the local, state, and federal levels and emphasized the need to reinforce or expand on those measures. The specific strengths and weaknesses of the public health response identified by local and state public health officials varied. Nonetheless, public health officials from all locations identified general lessons learned for public health preparedness. The lessons identified fall into three general categories: the benefits of planning and experience; the importance of effective communication, both among those involved in the response efforts and with the general public; and the critical importance of a strong public health infrastructure to serve as the foundation from which response efforts can be mounted for bioterrorism or other public health emergencies.

CDC was instrumental in supporting local and state efforts throughout the anthrax incidents, for example, by sending epidemic investigators into the field and providing laboratory expertise. DOD resources and expertise were also required to support several epicenters. CDC was challenged with the unfamiliar task of coordinating the extensive federal public health response efforts. Before the incidents began, CDC officials had recognized that the agency was not fully prepared to coordinate a major public health response effort and indeed had identified areas that needed improvement in testimony before Congress on the day before it confirmed the first case of inhalational anthrax in Florida. CDC officials have acknowledged that the agency did not perform as well as it would have liked during the incidents. The agency has taken steps to improve future performance, including creating the Office of Terrorism Preparedness and Emergency Response within the Office of the Director, building and staffing an emergency operations center, enhancing the agency's communication infrastructure, and developing and maintaining databases of information and expertise on the biological agents the federal government considers most likely to be used in a terrorist attack.

Agency Comments

We obtained comments on our draft report from DOD and HHS. (See apps. II and III.) DOD highlighted that lessons learned from its support of the public health response could aid in the development of expanded capabilities within the civilian sector to improve the nation's public health preparedness. DOD emphasized its capabilities that were vital to the success of the public health response, including environmental assessment, transportation of contaminated articles, laboratory testing, and cleanup of contaminated locations. The environmental cleanup was beyond the scope of this report.

HHS found the report to be informative and provided additional examples of actions taken to enhance national preparedness for bioterrorism and other public health emergencies. These examples included the establishment of the Office of Public Health Emergency Preparedness; the accelerated acquisition of antimicrobial drugs for the Strategic National Stockpile; and the expansion of basic and targeted research and upgrading of research facilities focused on the pathogens most likely to be used as bioterrorism agents.

DOD and HHS also made technical comments, which we incorporated where appropriate.

We are sending copies of this report to the Secretary of DOD, the Secretary of HHS, and other interested officials. We will also provide copies to others upon request. In addition, the report will be available at no charge on GAO's Web site at http://www.gao.gov.

If you or your staff have any questions about this report, please call me at (202) 512-7119. Another contact and key contributors are listed in appendix IV.

Sincerely yours,

Janet Heinrich
Director, Health Care—Public Health Issues

APPENDIX I: TIMELINE OF SELECTED KEY EVENTS IN THE ANTHRAX INCIDENTS

Date	**Events Occurring on That Date** ***Events Determined Retrospectively to Have Occurred on That Date* (in italics)**
Tuesday, 9/11/01	• Terrorist attack on World Trade Center and Pentagon prompts heightened epidemiologic surveillance activities in some areas.
Wednesday, 9/26/01 through Monday, 10/01/01	• *In New York (NY), two NBC employees, a* New York Post *employee, and the child of an ABC employee and in New Jersey (NJ), two U.S. Postal Service (USPS) employees, one from the West Trenton postal facility and one from Hamilton postal facility, seek medical attention for skin conditions.* • *In Florida, an American Media Inc. (AMI) employee is admitted to the hospital with a respiratory condition.*
Tuesday, 10/02/01	• The Centers for Disease Control and Prevention (CDC) issues a Health Alert Network (HAN) alert regarding preparedness for bioterrorism, acknowledging the public's concern about smallpox and anthrax and providing information about preventive measures. • *In Florida, a second AMI employee is admitted to the hospital, with a diagnosis of meningitis.*
Thursday, 10/04/01	• CDC and the Florida Department of Health announce confirmation of a case of inhalational anthrax. The infected person is an AMI employee, and the cause of the infection is unknown.
Friday, 10/05/01	• In Florida, an AMI employee becomes the first anthrax victim to die.
Sunday, 10/07/01	• In Florida, the AMI building is closed after anthrax spores are found.
Monday, 10/08/01	• In Florida, prophylaxis of AMI employees begins.
Wednesday, 10/10/01	• Because the source of the AMI employee's anthrax exposure is believed to have been a letter, USPS begins nationwide employee education on signs of anthrax exposure and procedures for handling mail to avoid anthrax infection.
Friday, 10/12/01	• In NY, the New York City Department of Health (NYCDOH) announces the confirmation of a case of cutaneous anthrax in an NBC employee. • USPS says that it will offer gloves and masks to all employees who handle mail.
Monday, 10/15/01	• On Capitol Hill, an employee opens a letter addressed to Senator Daschle thought to contain anthrax spores. People thought to be in the vicinity of the letter when it was opened are treated with ciprofloxacin, at the time the only drug approved for postexposure prophylaxis for anthrax. • In Florida, CDC confirms a second case of inhalational anthrax in an AMI employee. • In NY, NYCDOH announces a second case of cutaneous anthrax, in a child of an ABC employee.
Thursday, 10/18/01	• In the Washington, D.C., regional area (DC),[a] USPS reports that although it believes that the Daschle letter, which was processed at the Brentwood postal facility, was extremely well sealed and that there was a minute chance that anthrax spores escaped into the facility, it is testing the facility for anthrax contamination; quick tests are negative, other tests are sent to the laboratory. • In NJ, laboratory testing confirms cutaneous anthrax in two USPS employees, one from the West Trenton postal facility and one from the Hamilton postal facility.

Date	**Events Occurring on That Date** ***Events Determined Retrospectively to Have Occurred on That Date* (in italics)**
	• In NY, NYCDOH announces a third case of cutaneous anthrax, in a CBS employee. • In Florida, USPS closes two postal facilities contaminated with anthrax spores for cleaning. • In a telebriefing, the Director of CDC provides information about anthrax, including risk of exposure, availability of vaccines and antimicrobial medications, screening tests, symptoms, and what to do with suspicious mail and also explains CDC's role in the investigation. • CDC broadcasts part one of a live satellite and Web broadcast on anthrax for clinicians. • FDA announces that it has approved doxycycline for postexposure prophylaxis for anthrax. • *In DC, a USPS employee who works at the Brentwood postal facility seeks medical attention.*
Friday, 10/19/01	• In DC, a USPS employee who works at both the Brentwood postal facility and a Maryland postal facility is admitted to a hospital with suspected inhalational anthrax. • In NJ, the Hamilton and West Trenton postal facilities are closed, and the New Jersey Department of Health and Senior Services recommends that all USPS employees from both facilities receive prophylaxis. • In NJ, laboratory testing confirms cutaneous anthrax in a second USPS employee who works at the Hamilton postal facility. • In NY, NYCDOH announces a fourth case of cutaneous anthrax, in a *New York Post* employee.
Saturday, 10/20/01	• *In DC, a third USPS employee who works at the Brentwood postal facility is admitted to a hospital with a respiratory condition.*
Sunday, 10/21/01	• In DC, the USPS employee who worked at the Brentwood and Maryland postal facilities and was admitted to the hospital on 10/19/01 is confirmed to have inhalational anthrax. • In DC, the Brentwood and Maryland postal facilities, are closed. Evaluation and prophylaxis of employees begin. • In DC, a USPS employee who worked at the Brentwood postal facility and who initially sought medical attention on 10/18/01 is admitted to a hospital with suspected inhalational anthrax and becomes the second anthrax victim to die. • *In DC, a fourth USPS employee who worked at the Brentwood postal facility seeks medical attention at a hospital. His chest X-ray is initially determined to be normal, and he is discharged.*
Monday, 10/22/01	• In DC, the USPS employee who worked at the Brentwood postal facility and who sought medical attention on 10/21/01 and was discharged is admitted to the hospital with suspected inhalational anthrax, and becomes the third anthrax victim to die. • In DC, the USPS employee who was admitted to the hospital on 10/20/01 is confirmed to have inhalational anthrax. • In DC, prophylaxis is expanded to include all employees and visitors to nonpublic areas at the Brentwood postal facility. • CDC rebroadcasts part one of the live satellite and Web broadcast on anthrax for clinicians.

Date	**Events Occurring on That Date** ***Events Determined Retrospectively to Have Occurred on That Date* (in italics)**
Wednesday, 10/24/01	• In NY, USPS begins giving prophylaxis to employees at six New York City postal facilities where contaminated letters may have been processed.
Thursday, 10/25/01	• In DC, a State Department mail facility employee is called back to the hospital for admission; test taken the previous day is positive for inhalational anthrax. • In NY, NYCDOH announces a fifth case of cutaneous anthrax, in a second NBC employee. • CDC initiates daily telebriefings to provide updates on the anthrax incidents.
Saturday, 10/27/01	• In NY, NYCDOH announces the sixth case of cutaneous anthrax, in a second *New York Post* employee.
Sunday, 10/28/01	• In NJ, laboratory testing confirms inhalational anthrax in a USPS Hamilton employee who was admitted to a hospital with suspected inhalational anthrax on 10/19/01.
Monday, 10/29/01	• In NY, preliminary tests indicate anthrax in a hospital employee who was admitted with suspected inhalational anthrax on 10/28/01. The hospital where she works is temporarily closed, and NYCDOH recommends prophylaxis for hospital employees and visitors. • In NJ, laboratory testing confirms cutaneous anthrax in a woman who receives mail directly from the Hamilton facility. The woman originally sought medical attention on 10/18/01 and was admitted to the hospital on 10/22/01 for a skin condition. • In NJ, laboratory testing confirms a second case of inhalational anthrax, in a USPS Hamilton employee who initially sought medical attention on 10/16/01 and was admitted to the hospital on 10/18/01 with a respiratory condition.
Wednesday, 10/31/01	• In NY, the hospital employee becomes the fourth anthrax victim to die.[b]
Thursday, 11/01/01	• CDC broadcasts part two of the live satellite and Web broadcast on anthrax for clinicians.
Friday, 11/2/01	• In NY, NYCDOH announces the seventh case of cutaneous anthrax, in a third *New York Post* employee.
Wednesday, 11/21/01	• In Connecticut, an elderly woman, who was admitted to the hospital for dehydration on 11/16/01, becomes the fifth anthrax victim to die.[b] • The Connecticut Department of Public Health, in consultation with CDC, begins prophylaxis for USPS employees working in the Seymour and Wallingford postal facilities.
Friday, 12/21/01	• CDC expands the options for those on prophylaxis to include extending the duration of drug therapy and adding the anthrax vaccine.

Source: CDC, Connecticut Department of Public Health, District of Columbia Department of Health, FDA, Florida Department of Health, New Jersey Department of Health and Senior Services, NYCDOH, Office of the Attending Physician of the U.S. Congress, and USPS.

[a] The Washington, D.C., regional area includes Washington, D.C., Maryland, and Virginia.

[b] As of September 30, 2003, the source of exposure had not been confirmed.

INDEX

H

I

K

L

M

N

S

T

U

V

W